Epidemiology of

MONGOLISM

Epidemiology of **Mongolism**

Abraham M. Lilienfeld

with the assistance of

Charlotte H. Benesch

The Johns Hopkins Press, Baltimore

Manufactured in the United States of America

Library of Congress Catalog Card Number 78-82451

Standard Book Number 8018-1051-5

Acknowledgments

The author expresses his gratitude to the Joseph P. Kennedy, Jr., Foundation for the writing award which provided for the preparation of this review. He is also deeply grateful to Drs. Bernice H. Cohen and Morton L. Levin of the Department of Chronic Diseases, The Johns Hopkins School of Hygiene and Public Health, for their thorough review of the manuscript. This work was also supported in part by Research Career Award No. 5 K 06 GM 13,901 from the National Institute of General Medical Sciences, National Institutes of Health, Bethesda, Maryland.

Contents

Acknowledgments v

Chapter 1. *Background* 1
Mongolism 1
Epidemiology 9

Chapter 2. *Incidence* 15
General 15
Racial and Ethnic Groups 22
Maternal Age 27
Paternal Age 38
Grandparents' Agc 42
Birth Order 43

Chapter 3. *Distribution in Time and Space* 47
Clustering 47
Seasonal Distribution 56
General Comments 58

Chapter 4. *Maternal and Prenatal Factors* 59
Menstrual History 59
Reproductive Performance 59
Exposure to Ionizing Radiation 65
Maternal Ill Health during Pregnancy 68
Maternal Exposure to Fluorides in the Water Supply ... 69
Other Maternal Factors 70

Chapter 5. *Familial Aggregation and Twin Studies* 75
Familial Aggregation of Mongolism 75
Other Chromosomal Abnormalities in Families of Mongols 81
Offspring of Females with Mongolism 82
Twin Studies 82

Chapter 6. *The Association of Mongolism with Other Diseases* 85
Mongolism and Leukemia 85
Familial Aggregation of Mongolism and Leukemia 93
Mongolism and Thyroid Disease 94
Mongolism and Other Chromosomal Abnormalities 97
Mongolism and Other Diseases 98

Chapter 7. *Selected Characteristics of Mongols Including Mortality Experience* 99
Blood Groups 99
Biochemical Studies 100
Variability of Mongols 102
Mortality Experience 104

Chapter 8. *Etiological Hypotheses and Suggested Epidemiological Research* 107
Etiological Hypotheses 107
Suggested Epidemiological Research 111

References 115

Selected Bibliography 133

Index 143

List of Tables

Table 2–1. Summary of Studies on Incidence of Mongolism (per 1,000 Births), 1923–66. 16
Table 2–2. Frequency Distribution of Reports of Incidence Rates of Mongolism (per 1,000 Births). 19
Table 2–3. Summary of Reports on Chromosomal Studies of Spontaneous and Induced Abortions, 1960–66. 20
Table 2–4. Incidence of Mongolism (per 1,000 Live Births) by Continent of Origin, Western Jerusalem, Israel, 1964–66. 23

Table 2–5. Incidence Rates of Mongolism Standardized for Maternal Age for Selected Centers in Various Countries. 24
Table 2–6. Negro Mongols Found in Literature Survey. 25
Table 2–7. Percentage Frequencies of the Major Chromosomal Anomalies in Down's Syndrome. 26
Table 2–8. Summary of Selected Studies on Incidence Rates of Mongolism (per 1,000 Births) by Maternal Age, 1923–64. 27
Table 2–9. Summary of Selected Studies of Relative Frequency of Mongolism (per cent Mongols/per cent Controls) by Maternal Age. 29
Table 2–10. Theoretical Maternal Age Distributions of 2 Populations, Demonstrating the Movement of the Early Down's Maternal Age Peak with Actual Age-Specific Incidence Rates Held Constant. 32
Table 2–11. Estimation of the Proportion of Maternal Age-Independent and Age-Dependent Mongols. 34
Table 2–12. Estimation of the Expected Number of Total and Maternal Age-Independent and Age-Dependent Mongols. 34
Table 2–13. The Cumulative Expected Number and per cent of Mongol Births (from Older to Younger Maternal Ages) by Maternal Age Estimated for U.S. Live Births, 1960. 35
Table 2–14. Chromosomal Findings on Patients with Down's Syndrome—Pooled Data from Several Studies. 35
Table 2–15. Frequencies and Proportions of Inherited and Sporadic Translocations. 36
Table 2–16. Mean Interval between Marriage and First Birth for 96 Mothers of Children with Down's Syndrome, Grouped According to Whether the First-born Child Is Affected or Not. 36
Table 2–17. Duration of Marriage in Years by Age of Mother at Birth of Child. 37
Table 2–18. Mongolism Cases by Parental Ages, Upstate New York, 1950–62. 39
Table 2–19. Paternal Age Distribution and Relative Incidence, after Exclusion of Maternal Age Effect. 40

Table 2–20. Matched Pair Analysis of Paternal Age with Maternal Age Controlled (Paired *t* Test). 40
Table 2–21. Relative Incidence of Down's Syndrome According to Paternal Age, with Maternal Age Controlled. 41
Table 2–22. Probability of a Mongol (per 1,000 Births) by Mother's Age at Birth of Mongol and Grandmother's Age at Birth of the Mother. 42
Table 2–23. Maternal Age at Birth of 1,282 Patients with Down's Syndrome, by Grandmaternal Age at Birth of Mothers. 43
Table 2–24. Mongolism Occurrence Rates per 1,000 Live Births by Age of Mother and Birth Order, Lower Michigan, 1950–64. 44
Table 2–25. Distribution of Live-Birth Rank, after Exclusion of Maternal Age Effect. 44
Table 2–26. Relative Incidence of Down's Syndrome and Other Mental Defects for Each Rank in the Live-Birth Order, with Maternal Age Controlled. 45
Table 3–1. Summary of Studies on Temporo-Spatial Clustering of Mongolism in Different Geographical Areas. 49
Table 3–2. Numbers of Cases and Incidences of Infectious Hepatitis (per 100,000 of Population) and of Births of Children 9 Months Later with Down's Syndrome (per 100,000 Live Births) for the Eastern and Western Areas of Melbourne, Australia. 53
Table 3–3. Annual Incidence Rate (per 1,000 Births) for Mongols and Expected Numbers Based on Total Rate for Births, South Dakota, 1954–61. 53
Table 3–4. Proportion of Pairs of Cases and Mongolism Not More Than 4 Kilometers Apart, 1950–54 and 1955–64. 54
Table 3–5. Annual and Over-all Monthly Incidence of Down's Syndrome (per 100,000 Live Births) for the Lower Peninsula of Michigan, 1950–64. 55
Table 3–6. Relationship between Monthly Temperature 8 Months before Birth and Frequency of Mongol Births. 58
Table 4–1. Menstrual History of Mothers of Children with Down's Syndrome and of Control Children. 60
Table 4–2. Interval between Birth of Mongoloid or Control and Preceding Birth, by 2 Age Groups. 61

Table 4–3. Observed and Expected Numbers of Pregnancies for Mothers of Mongols in Specific Maternal Age Periods by Age at Birth of Mongol. 63
Table 4–4. Fetal Losses per 100 Pregnancies in Mothers of Mongols and in Control Mothers. 64
Table 4–5. Pregnancy Wastage in Mothers of Children with Down's Syndrome and in Mothers of Controls by Maternal Age and by Time Relationship to Index Child. 65
Table 4–6. Distribution of the Interval Free from Pregnancy before the Births of Infants with Down's Syndrome and Controls Matched by Sex, Year of Birth, Maternal Age, and Live-Birth Rank. 66
Table 4–7. Summary of Parental Diagnostic, Fluoroscopic and Therapeutic Radiation (One or More Exposures), Interview, and Medical Records Prior to Birth of the Index Child. 67
Table 4–8. Frequency of Mongolism in Cities of 10,000–100,000 Population, Illinois, January 1, 1950–December 31, 1956. 70
Table 4–9. Observed and Expected Positive Thyroid Antibody Tests in Mothers of Children with Down's Syndrome in Relation to Maternal Age at Birth of the Propositus. . . 71
Table 4–10. Frequency of Positive Test for Thyroid Antibody and Other Characteristics of Mothers of Aneuploid Children and Controls. 72
Table 4–11. Marital and Reproductive History of Mothers of Children with Down's Syndrome and of Control Children. . . 73
Table 5–1. Relative Prevalence of Down's Syndrome in Sibs of Index Patients and in General Population. 76
Table 5–2. Comparison of Observed and Expected Number of Affected Sibs According to Mother's Age at Birth of Index Patient. 77
Table 5–3. Increased Risk of Having a Second Child with Mongolism. 77
Table 5–4. Distribution of Chromosomal Abnormalities in Several Series of Patients with Down's Syndrome by Maternal Ages at Parturition and by Type and Frequency of Translocation. 78

Table 5–5. Distribution of Mongol Twins from Summary of Case Reports. 83
Table 5–6. Summary of Index Cases in Terms of Zygosity and Concordance. 84
Table 6–1. Summary of Studies Showing Frequency of Mongols among Cases of Leukemia and a Comparison Group. . . 86
Table 6–2. Summary of Studies Showing Frequency of Leukemia among Mongols and a Comparison Group or Expected Frequency Based on Mortality Experience. 88
Table 6–3. Observed Versus Expected Number of Deaths Due to Leukemia in an Estimated Population of Pennsylvania Mongols, 1955–60. 90
Table 6–4. Comparison of Age- and Sex-Specific Leukemia Death Rates of the Institutionalized Mongol Population of Pennsylvania with Those of the General Pennsylvania Population. 90
Table 6–5. Comparison by Age and Sex of Observed Versus Expected Number of Deaths Due to Leukemia and Other Neoplasms Occurring among the Institutionalized Population of Mongols, Pennsylvania, 1945–49. . . 91
Table 6–6. Congenital Cytogenetic Disorders and Leukemia–Lymphoma. 93
Table 6–7. Case Reports of Aggregation of Congenital Chromosomal Abnormalities and Leukemia in Families. 94
Table 6–8. Thyroid Autoantibodies in Winnipeg and Seattle Females. 96
Table 6–9. Thyroid Autoantibodies in Mothers of Down's Syndrome Children Compared to Control Females. 97
Table 6–10. Frequency of Down's Syndrome in Patients with Hirschsprung's Disease. 98
Table 7–1. Summary of Findings of Studies of Biochemical Characteristics of Mongols. 101
Table 7–2. Distribution of Australia Antigen in Patients and U.S. Normals. 103
Table 7–3. Summary of Studies of Survivorship Experience of Mongols by Number of Years after Birth. 104
Table 7–4. Mortality in 1,236 Patients with Down's Syndrome, by Age. 105

Table 7–5. Observed and Expected Number of Deaths among Mongols by Cause of Death. 105
Table 8–1. Partition of Causes of Down's Syndrome. 109

List of Figures

Figure 1–1. Karyotype of a Normal Female. 3
Figure 1–2. Karyotype of a Regular Female Mongol Showing Trisomy of Chromosome Number 21. 4
Figure 1–3. Nondisjunction at First Meiotic Division. 5
Figure 1–4. Nondisjunction at Second Meiotic Division. 6
Figure 1–5. Normal Meiosis. 7
Figure 1–6. Diagram to Show the Origin of the 13–15/21 Translocation and Its Mode of Inheritance. 8
Figure 1–7. The Production of Chromosome Mosaics by Mitotic (Chromatid) Nondisjunction during Cleavage of a Normal Zygote. 11
Figure 1–8. Representation of Origin of Standard Trisomic Mongolism by Mitotic Error in Trisomic Zygotes. 12
Figure 2–1. Incidence Rates of Mongolism by Maternal Age from Selected Studies, 1923–64. 28
Figure 2–2. Relative Frequency of Mongolism (per cent Mongols/ per cent Controls) by Maternal Age. 30
Figure 2–3. Distribution of All Births and Mongol Births by Maternal Age, Victoria, Australia, 1942–57. 31
Figure 2–4. Theoretical Distributions of General Populations *A* and *B* with Corresponding Distributions of Cases of Down's Syndrome Using the Same Age-Specific Incidence Rates on Each Population. 33
Figure 3–1. Annual Incidence of Mongol Births Adjusted for Annual Variations in the Quinquennial Age Distribution of All Parturient Mothers in the General Population, Victoria, Australia, 1942–57. 51
Figure 3–2. Annual Incidence of Infective Hepatitis (per Million) Followed 9 Months Later by Births (per 100,000 Live Births) of Children with Down's Syndrome, Victoria, Australia, 1952–64. 52

Etiological Model A 110

Etiological Model B 111

1:

Background

To arrive at an understanding of the epidemiology of mongolism and to be able to consider its future research potential requires some familiarity with the general concepts of mongolism and epidemiology, as well as with the technical terminology associated with both. Obviously it would be neither possible nor necessary to review these in detail here, and therefore the general references include several recently published books and papers to which the interested reader is referred. However, it does appear worth-while and desirable to review selectively those areas having special relevance to the particular issues and problems discussed in this book.

Mongolism

"Furfuraceous idiocy" was a description given by Séquin in 1846 to a specific type of mental retardation. Many today still consider this a most accurate description of the physical characteristics of the mongoloid growth deficiency. In 1867, J. Langdon Down, influenced by the racial hypothesis, described this mental deficiency syndrome as "mongolism." Through the years the racial implication of the term mongolism has been responsible for suggestions to adopt such terms as Down's syndrome or Down's anomaly. In spite of these efforts, the term mongolism continues to be used extensively in the literature and has been selected for use in this review. From 1846 until 1959 countless etiological hypotheses had been considered and examined but almost all were eventually rejected when, in 1959, Lejeune, Gautier, and Turpin (1959*b*) demonstrated what had been suspected earlier, that mongols usually have a chromosomal anomaly (Bleyer; Penrose, 1939; Waardenburg). These investigators observed that most of the cells of the examined patients had 47 chromosomes instead of the usual 46 (Figure 1–1, Figure 1–2). This extra chromosome is found in what is classified as chromosome pair 21 and has therefore been responsible for the descriptive term trisomy 21 for this condition. Observations from chromosomal studies in other species have demonstrated that such trisomies develop as a result of nondisjunction, a failure of homologous chromosomes to separate during the anaphase stage of cell division (Bridges; Sturtevant). Nondisjunction occurring during the first or second meiotic division is illustrated in Figures 1–3 and 1–4 in contrast to normal meiosis (Figure 1–5).

Shortly after the discovery of trisomy 21 it became evident that not all cases of mongolism were characterized by trisomy. In 1960, Polani, Ford, Briggs, and Clarke observed a mongol girl with only 46 chromosomes. It was postulated that a reciprocal translocation had occurred between 2 chromosomal groups, one of which was probably group 21. Specifically a break had occurred in one of the chromosomes and the broken part was transferred and fused with one of the chromosomes of another group. The fertilized ovum containing an extra piece of chromosome number 21 attached to another chromosome produces the same clinical consequence of mongolism as in trisomy 21; this mechanism is illustrated in Figure 1–6. Other ways by which translocations can occur have been postulated, and from various cytogenetic surveys of mongols it has been estimated that about 2 to 3 per cent of mongols are translocation mongols (Brøgger, Mohr, *et al.*; Cowie, 1966; Hamerton; Penrose & Smith).

The importance of translocation mongolism is that the translocated chromosome is carried by a normal person and passed through several generations (offspring number 3 in Figure 1–6); this is one of the major reasons for the familial occurrence of mongolism.

A third cytological type of mongolism is mosaic mongolism. In this condition certain types of cells contain the extra chromosome but the remaining cells have the normal number of chromosomes. Thus, the organism is composed of a mixture of cells with different numbers of chromosomes. Mosaics can arise from a normal zygote with 46 chromosomes as a result of nondisjunction during mitosis (Figure 1–7), or they can arise from an abnormal zygote with trisomy due to

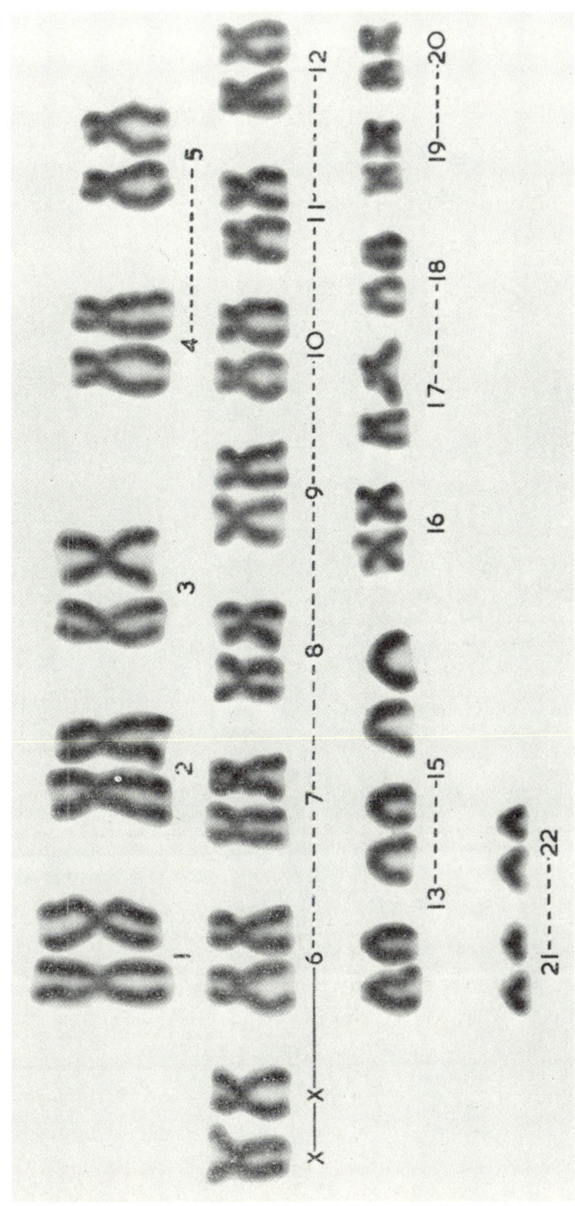

Figure 1–1: Karyotype of a Normal Female (*from: Ford*).

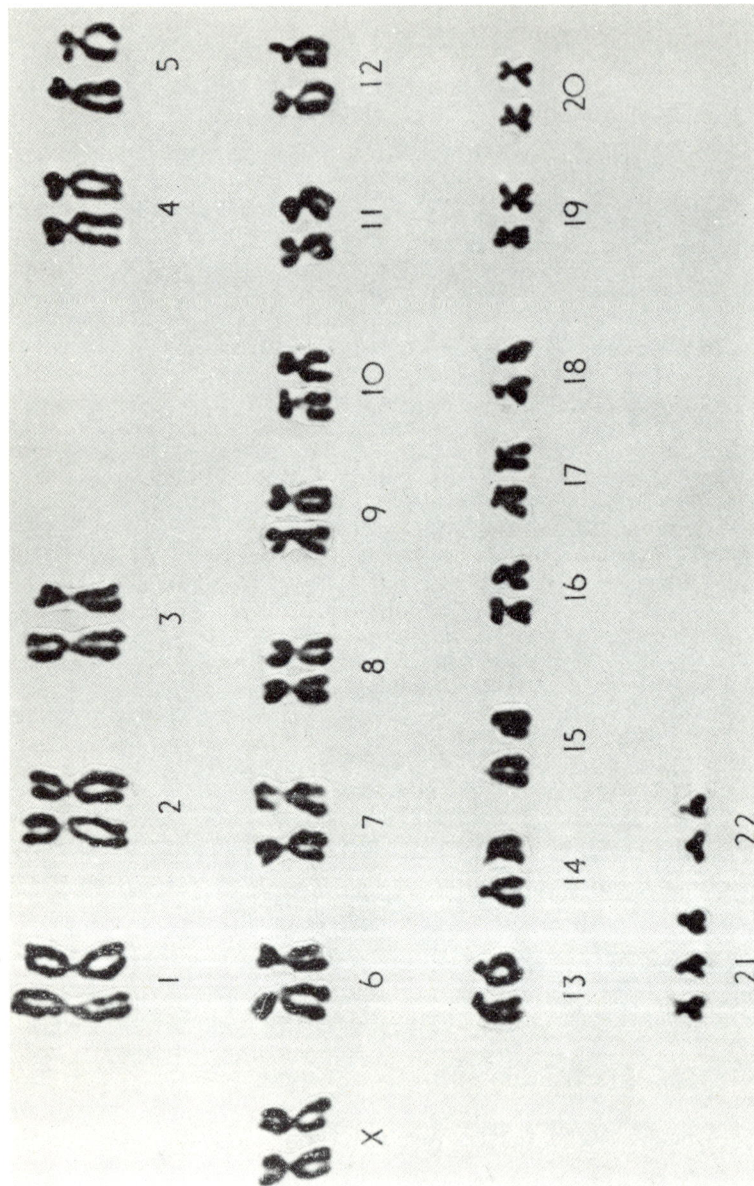

Figure 1–2. Karyotype of a Regular Female Mongol Showing Trisomy of Chromosome Number 21 (*from: Hamerton*).

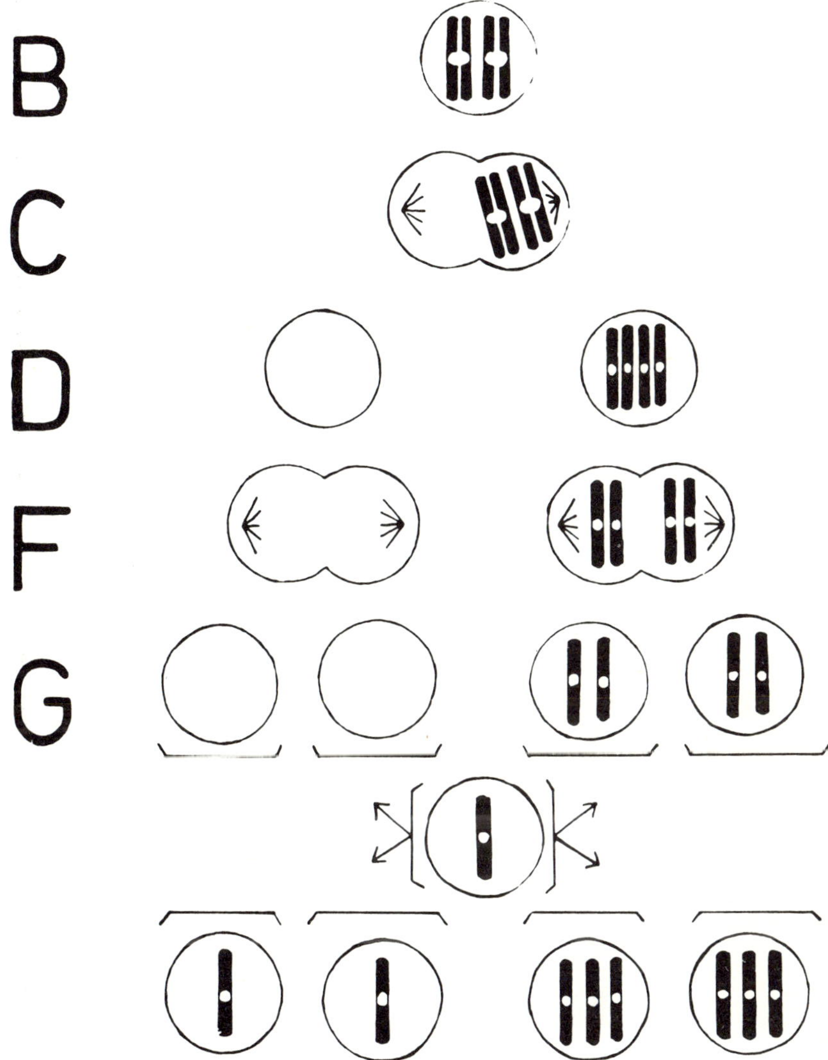

Figure 1–3. Nondisjunction at First Meiotic Division (*from: Robson*).

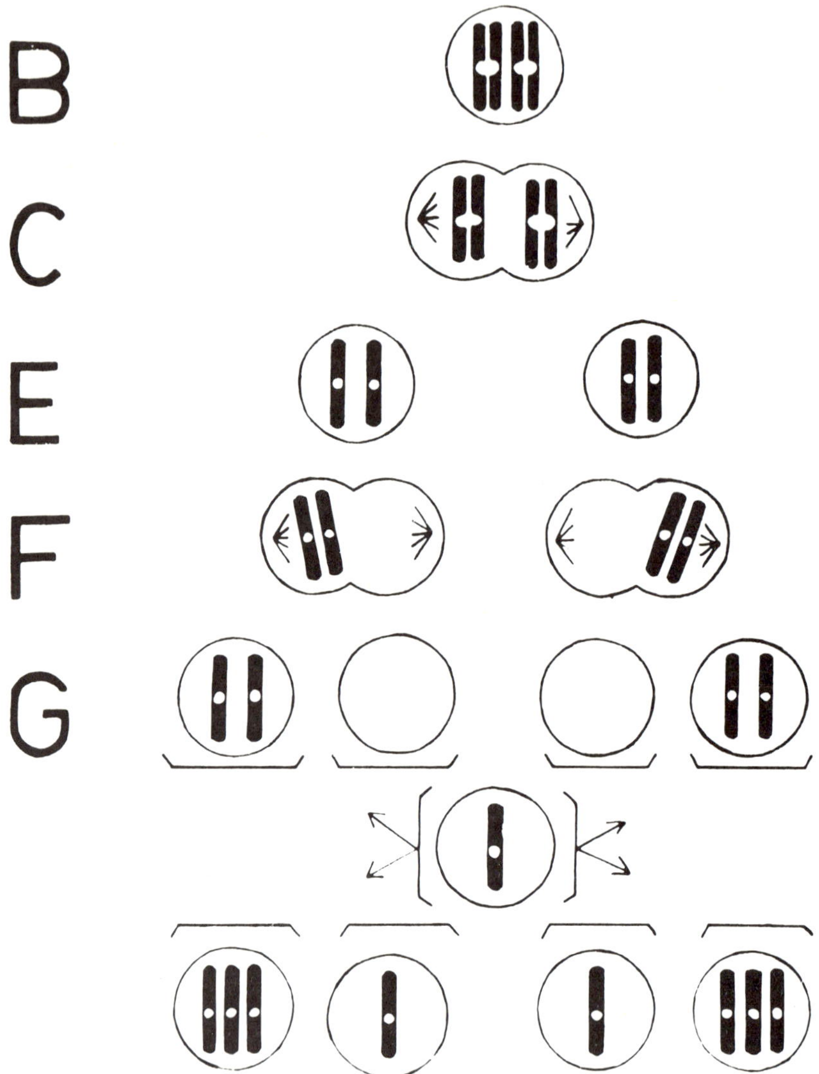

Figure 1–4. Nondisjunction at Second Meiotic Division (*from: Robson*).

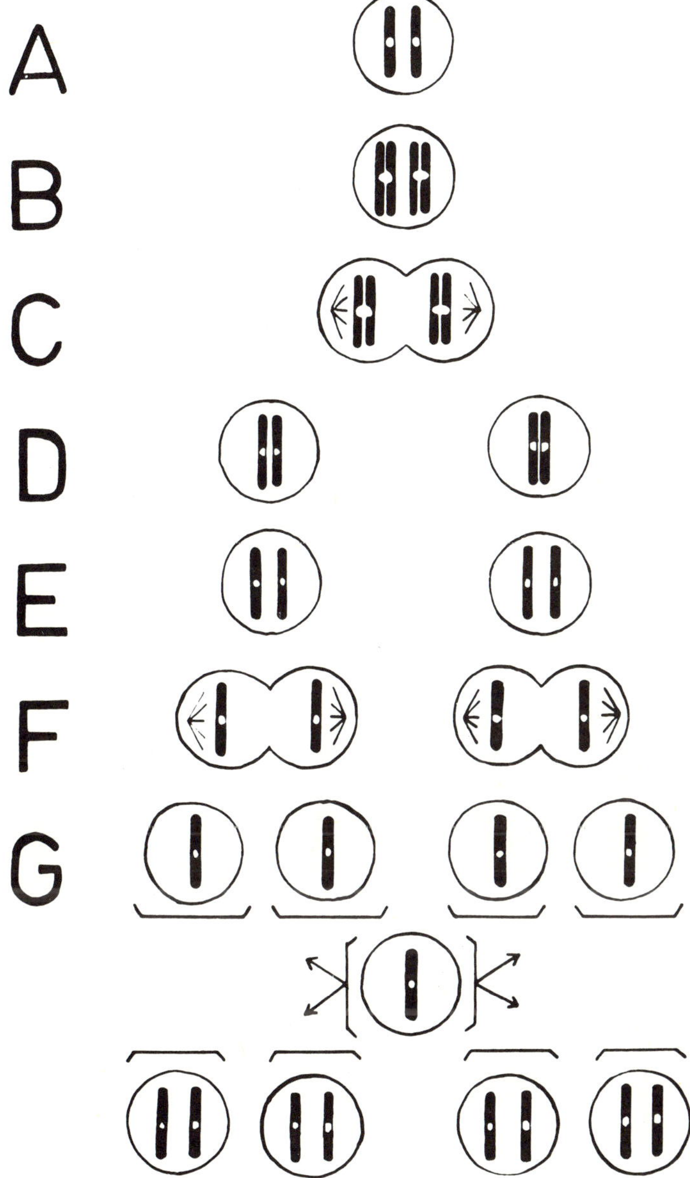

Figure 1–5. Normal Meiosis (*from: Robson*).

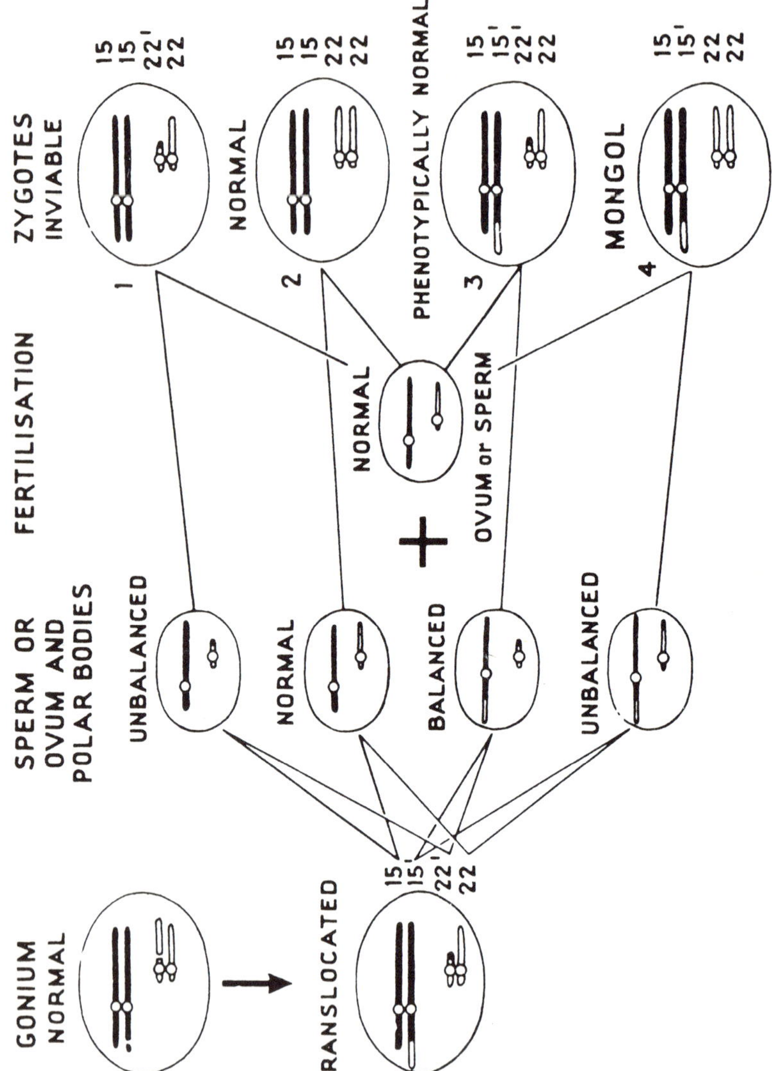

Figure 1–6. Diagram to Show the Origin of the 13–15/21 Translocation and Its Mode of Inheritance (*from: Miller & Dill*).

(Figure 1–6 Continued)

Note: This diagram was originally presented by Polani in 1960. Chromosome 22 in the original diagram is now classified as 21 and it is now recognized that the small fusion product is lost soon after the translocation occurs. For illustration, the translocation is shown as having occurred in a spermatogonium or oogonium. In the latter case, only one of the meiotic products becomes a functional gamete; the others become polar bodies. If the translocation originated earlier in development, the change would be propagated at each mitosis and more gonia would be affected in the same way. The exact positions of breakage cannot be defined and the points indicated have been chosen arbitrarily.

Offspring: 1 is a chromosomally unbalanced and presumably inviable zygote; 2 is normal, phenotypically and chromosomally; 3 is a chromosomally balanced phenotypically normal carrier; he is chromosomally distinct and will produce the same types of gametes and offspring as the affected parent; 4 is a mongol.

---

the loss of the extra chromosome during mitosis (Figure 1–8). The available surveys indicate that about 2 per cent of mongols are chromosomal mosaics (Cowie, 1966; Smith).

The importance of mosaicism in the total picture of mongolism is probably greater than this frequency indicates. It is theoretically possible that normal mothers of trisomic mongols may be chromosomal mosaics and that the abnormal chromosomal cells are in the ovarian tissue. Thus, the ova produced by such individuals contain trisomic cells and result in trisomic offspring. This type of mosaicism would not be detectable by cytological studies of the usual somatic tissues. Penrose and Smith, using dermatoglyphic surveys, estimated that about 10 per cent of normal-appearing mothers of mongols are chromosomal mosaics; they state that this could also occur in the fathers of the mongols and estimate this frequency at about 1 per cent.

Epidemiology

Epidemiology is defined as the study of the distribution of a disease in a population and of the factors influencing this distribution. Thus, the epidemiologist is interested in the distribution of disease by age, sex, race, urban-rural areas, geography, season, occupation, and other population characteristics. Essentially, he is concerned with 2 aspects: (1) differences in the frequency of the disease in different situations, and (2) characteristics of those who have the disease as compared to those who do not. This information is helpful both in suggesting etiological hypotheses and in testing etiological hypotheses developed from other scientific disciplines.

In describing the frequency of disease, 2 general types of rates are used, incidence and prevalence rates, which are defined as follows:

$$\text{(a) Incidence rate per 1,000 births} = \frac{\text{Number of cases of mongolism that occur during a certain period of time}}{\text{Number of births}} \times 1{,}000$$

These incidence rates can also be expressed in per cent, i.e., per 100 births. Reports in the literature show that investigators select and use different denominators, such as total births (live and stillbirths) or live births only and therefore the rates vary slightly depending on the type of denominator.

$$\text{(b) Prevalence rate per 1,000} = \frac{\text{Number of cases of mongols existing at a specified time}}{\text{Average number of persons in population at a specified time}} \times 1{,}000$$

It is important to note that the incidence rate provides a direct measure of the probability of developing a disease and therefore is the preferred type of measure. Prevalence rates are particularly useful in assessing the need for services; however, differences or changes in these rates may also provide a lead for further studies. The usefulness of prevalence rates is limited however, because they are related not only to the incidence but also to the duration of the disease. Prevalence is an indication of the balance between the development of new cases in the population and the withdrawal of cases because of death. In view of the relatively high death rates among mongols, prevalence of mongols at any given time is a distorted reflection of incidence.

These rates—incidence and prevalence—can be computed separately for the various forms of mongolism, for each sex, for different age groups, for separate maternal age groups, order of birth, urban and rural sections of the population, different countries, or for any population group or subgroup where the appropriate numerator and denominator figures are known.

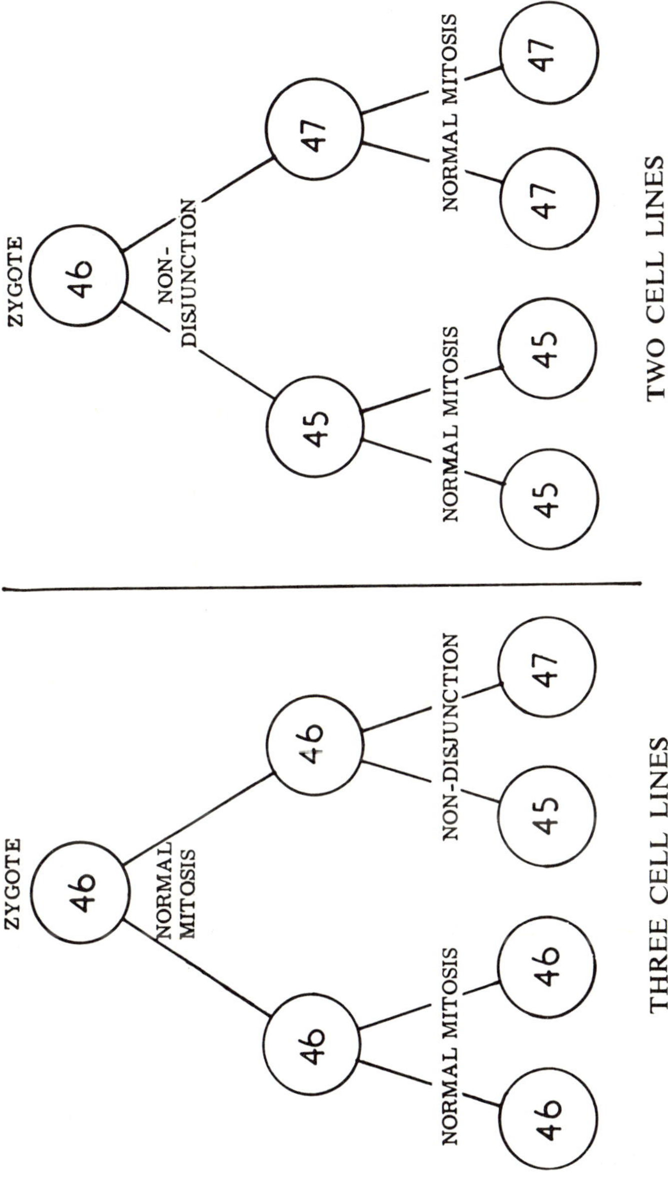

Figure 1–7. The Production of Chromosome Mosaics by Mitotic (Chromatid) Nondisjunction during Cleavage of a Normal Zygote (*from: Harnden*).

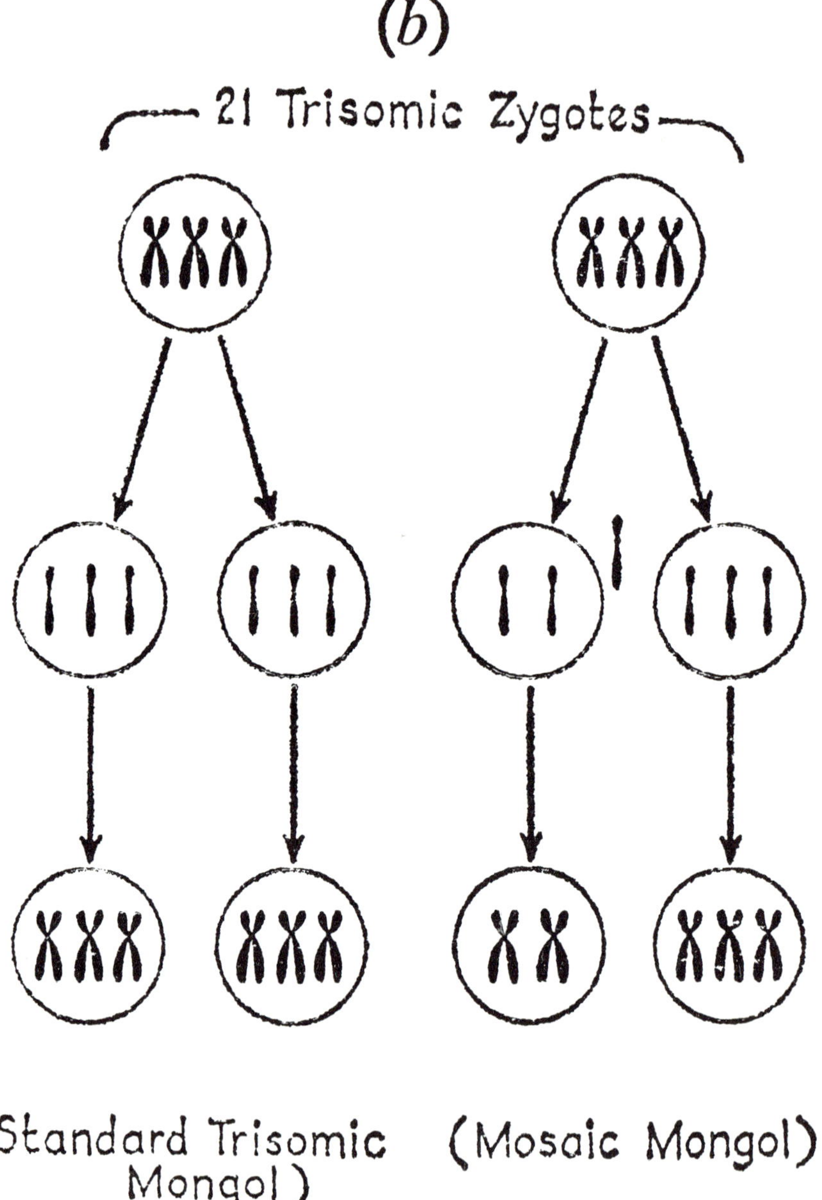

Figure 1–8. Representation of Origin of Standard Trisomic Mongolism by Mitotic Error in Trisomic Zygotes (*from: Penrose & Smith*).

There are 2 types of epidemiological studies which will be referred to here—retrospective and prospective studies. In retrospective studies, the investigator selects those with a disease and determines the frequency of past events in which he is interested. This frequency is compared with that of a control group of individuals for whom information is obtained in a similar manner. If the frequency of selected events is higher in the case than in the control group, an association is said to exist between the disease and the selected past events. An example of this type of approach is the study of histories of lifetime exposure to ionizing radiation among mothers of mongols as compared to a control group (Sigler, Lilienfeld, *et al.*, 1965*a*).

In a prospective study, the investigator selects persons who have the characteristic of etiological interest and a group which does not. He then follows these 2 groups and determines the frequency of the disease that develops. For example, if one is interested in studying the relationship between ionizing radiation and mongolism in this manner, one could select a group of women who have been exposed to therapeutic radiation for various reasons and a group which has not. One would then follow these women through their subsequent pregnancies to determine the incidence of mongol births. More detailed descriptions of these 2 types of studies, as well as a discussion of their advantages and disadvantages, can be found in publications by MacMahon, Pugh, and Ipsen; and Lilienfeld, Pedersen, and Dowd.

2:

Incidence

General

There has been a prolific accumulation of reports on the incidence of mongolism among the newborn and a summary of these reports representing some 34 studies is presented in Table 2–1. It includes the year of study, geographical area, method of ascertainment of mongols, and the number of births and mongols upon which the incidence rates are based.

The methods used to determine the number of newborn mongols have ranged from a retrospective review of hospital records to an actual examination of the newborn during a prescribed period of time. We note in viewing Table 2–1 that the majority of the studies represent a retrospective review of hospital records. The errors inherent in this approach are obvious; hospitals with pediatricians who have a particular interest in mongolism would be more sensitive to such a diagnosis and would probably be more disposed to record it on routine records. In addition, a large proportion of the reports come from individual hospitals, where selective admission policies might have inadvertently favored mothers with certain characteristics affecting the incidence of mongolism, e.g., if a hospital selectively admits younger mothers the incidence will be low, for as will be demonstrated later, maternal age is significantly related to incidence. The reported rates range from 0.32 to 3.4 per 1,000 births; the frequency distribution of these rates is presented in Table 2–2.

Table 2–1. Summary of Studies on Incidence of Mongolism (per 1,000 Births), 1923–66

Investigator and year of report	Years of study	Geographical area	Method of ascertainment	Number of births	Number of mongols	Incidence rate per 1,000
Malpas (1937)	1923–32	Liverpool, England	Obstetrical records and questionnaire to parents.	13,964 (total)	18	1.29
Øster (1953)	1923–49	Rigshospitalet, Seeland Neighbouring Islands, Denmark	Traced through diagnosis, card-indices and birth records in 2 departments.	84,072 (live)	71	0.84
Jenkins (1933)	1926–31	Presbyterian Hospital, Chicago	All newborns examined and diagnosed by physician.	3,818	6	1.6
Beidelman (1945)	1930–44 (?)	Boston Lying-In Hospital	Hospital records.	about 12,352	42	3.4
Stevenson, Worcester, & Rice (1950)	1930–41	Boston Lying-In Hospital	Obstetric records.	29,024 (total)	15	0.52
Hug (1951)	1930–49	Zürich St. Gallen, Switzerland	Not reported.	67,645 (total)	130	1.9
Parker (1950)	1939–48	Gallinger Municipal Hospital, Washington, D.C.	Obstetric records with pediatric follow-up.	27,931 (live)	32	1.15
Record & Smith (1955)	1942–52	Birmingham, England	Records of Maternity Hospital, Children's Hospital, Public Health Dept. records, local health authority, and data from other study	231,619 (total)	252	1.09
Beolchini, Bariatti, & Morganti (1962)	1942–57	Provincial Maternal Institute of Milan	Not reported.	54,482 (total)	91	1.7
Collmann & Stoller (1963*a*)	1942–57	Victoria, Australia	All available medical and educational facilities contacted by personal visits or letters, review of death certificates.	780,168 (live)	1,134	1.45
Harris & Steinberg (1954)	1944–50	St. Marys Hospital, Rochester, Minn.	Physical examination during first 6 days of life, majority of examinations by authors.	8,716 (live)	11	1.26
Pleydell (1957)	1944–55	Northamptonshire, England	All medical and educational facilities including local health authorities.	52,729 (total)	86	1.63

Table 2–1. Continued

Investigator and year of report	Years of study	Geographical area	Method of ascertainment	Number of births	Number of mongols	Incidence rate per 1,000
Landtman (1948)	1945–48	University College Hospital, London	Obstetric and pediatric records.	3,593 (total)	4	1.11
Carter & MacCarthy (1951)	Varying periods in different hospitals.	London, England	Hospital records of 12 maternity units and hospitals.	71,521 (total)	107	1.5
Kurland (1958)	1945–54	Rochester, Minn.	Diagnosed at birth and subsequently confirmed at later examination.	14,200 (live)	14	1.0
McIntosh, Merrit, *et al.* (1954)	1946–53	Sloane Hospital for Women, N.Y. City	Each infant had careful examination by pediatrician; 6 and 12 months follow-up examination.	5,964 (total)	11	1.8
Gentry, Parkhurst, & Bulin (1959)	1948–55	N.Y. State (exclusive of N.Y. City)	Birth and death certificates.	1,242,744 (live)	392	0.32
Buchan (1962)	1948–59	Newcastle-upon-Tyne, England	Review of pediatric notes, register of defective children death certificates, hospital records.	61,821 (total)	92	1.48
Stark & Mantel (1967)	1950–64	Lower Michigan	Birth certificates, state institutions, hospitals, and public schools.	2,722,774 (live)	2,432	0.89
Leck (1966)	1950–65	Birmingham, England	Birth records, hospital admission returns, death certificates, necropsy reports, local health authorities.	316,954 (live)	513	1.62
McDonald (1961)	1952–55	Watford, England	Examination of newborn by physician.	3,179 (live)	6	1.9
Lunn (1959)	1953–58	Glasgow, Scotland	Not reported.	128,000 (approx. total)	130	1.02
Hedberg, Holmdahl, *et al.* (1963)	1954–58	Gothenberg, Sweden	Follow-up of pregnant women who visited a prenatal care center in Gothenberg and pediatric records.	3,000 (total)	4	1.33

Table 2–1. Concluded

Investigator and year of report	Years of study	Geographical area	Method of ascertainment	Number of births	Number of mongols	Incidence rate per 1,000
Renwick, Miller, & Paterson (1964)	1955	British Columbia, Canada	Registry for handicapped children and vital records.	34,138 (live)	50	1.46
Babbott & Ingalls (1962)	1955–60	Pennsylvania	Review of hospital records of newborns.	25,760 (live)	26	1.01
Brewis, Poskanzer, *et al.* (1966)	1955–61	Carlisle, Cumberland, England	Review of all medical records in community, including physician records.	8,528 (live)	10	1.2
Halevi (1967)	1959–60	Israel	Review of obstetric records in hospitals.	90,792 (total)	97	1.07
Turner (1963)	1960	Pennsylvania	Estimation from death certificates and records of mongols in institutions.	243,118 (live)	304	1.25
Hall (1964)	1961–62	Southern Sweden	Pediatrician's reports of all suspect cases of mongolism and cytological follow-up of 90 per cent and clinical examination.	25,038 (total)	38	1.52
Stevenson, Johnston, *et al.* (1966)	Approximately 1961–64	24 hospitals in 16 countries	Study from a fixed date in each hospital, information and detailed description by physician obtained on each malformation in every still and live birth over 28 weeks of gestation. Physician described each malformation.	416,695 (total)	347	0.83
Spellman (1966)	1962–63	Cork City and County, Ireland	Survey of physicians and midwives and maternity hospitals.	15,517 (total)	27	1.7
Robinson & Puck (1967)	1962–66	Denver, Colo. (2 hospitals)	Chromosomal analysis of newborn in whom mongolism was clinically suspected.	11,646 (total)	13	1.12
Davidenkova, Shtil'bans, *et al.* (1964)	Not reported	Leningrad	Not reported.	131,634 (total)	134	1.02
Brochier (1947)	Not reported	Hospital of Croix-Rousse	Not reported.	15,600 (total)	18	1.15

Note: Total includes live births and stillbirths.

Table 2–2. Frequency Distribution of Reports of Incidence Rates of Mongolism (per 1,000 Births)

Incidence rate (per 1,000 births)	Number of reports
<1.0	5
1.0–1.4	18
1.5–1.9	10
2.0+	1
Total	34

When one considers the element of variability in the diagnostic criteria, in the record keeping, in maternal characteristics, etc., in these reported studies, it is surprising to find that the incidence rates show as high a degree of uniformity as they do. The two reports where the incidence of mongolism was determined concurrently were by Hall and by McIntosh, Merrit, Richards, Samuels, and Bellows; the first showed an incidence rate of 1.5 and the latter, 1.8 per 1,000.

The reports are arranged as nearly as possible in chronological sequence in an attempt to provide some idea of possible frequency changes in mongolism over time. Although these data may well be too crude and variable to discern any trend (if one exists), it was felt that any marked changes in incidence would be apparent. These data do not suggest such a trend, but do not rule out the possibility that slight or moderate changes in incidence rates have occurred.

The reported incidence rates are based on the determination of the presence of mongolism at the time of birth. In evaluating incidence rates, either in general or in terms of specific subgroups of the population, there are other considerations that must be taken into account. Over the past several years, the results of chromosomal studies of abortions, both spontaneous and induced, have been reported (Makino, Kikuchi, *et al.*) and in general have shown a high frequency of chromosomal changes. The examination of about 261 spontaneously aborted fetuses reveals that about 28 per cent had chromosomal abnormalities, which is much greater than the frequency observed among live-born infants. A review of these papers indicates that about 4 per cent (10 out of 261) of the spontaneous abortions have trisomy 21 (Table 2–3); this proportion is obviously higher than the frequency of mongolism among newborn.

Table 2–3. Summary of Reports on Chromosomal Studies of Spontaneous and Induced Abortions, 1960–66

Investigator and year of report	Years of study	Study method	Abortions			
			Total	Number examined	Number of trisomy 21	Number other trisomic types
Makino, Kikuchi, *et al.* (1962)	1960–61	Random samplings from different organs of legally aborted fetuses from several hospitals of private facilities located in different districts in the city of Sapporo.	135	127	0	0
Szulman (1965)	1961–62	All available material from spontaneous abortions except infected ones. Department of Pathology, Boston Lying-In Hospital and Harvard Medical School (amnion chosen to grow in culture).	75	25	3	E–2 C–1
Carr (1963)	1962	Chromosome studies in cells grown from tissue obtained from 35 spontaneous abortions, 6 stillborn infants. Aborted specimens were unselected except if there was good reason to doubt spontaneity.	35	35	1	E–1 D–3
Carr (1967)	1962–65	South Western Ontario: collected in 2½ years (1) spontaneously aborted embryos, fetuses, and sacs which were successfully grown in culture; (2) spontaneous abortions which failed to grow in culture; (3) induced abortions, ectopic pregnancies, and stillborn infants.	400	227	6 (1 with abnormal G)	A–1 B–1 C–2 D–6 E–9 F–1
Clendenin & Benirschke (1963)	1963	Department of Obstetrics and Gynecology and Department of Pathology, Mary Hitchcock Memorial Hospital, Hanover, N.H. All tissue from spontaneous abortions and previable deliveries treated in the hospital. Usually these were incomplete abortions.	140 conclusions of pregnancy 18 spontaneous abortions	10	0	E–1
Waxman, Arakaki, & Smith (1967)	1964–66	All consecutive abortions from a large maternity hospital were examined for chromosome abnormalities (Hawaii). Specimens screened by pathologist. 149 were spontaneous abortions.	149	25	0	E–4 F–1

Table 2–3. Continued

Investigator and year of report	Years of study	Study method	Abortions: Total	Number examined	Number of trisomy 21	Number other trisomic types
Thiede & Salm (1964)	Not reported	51 specimens came from emergency department or gynecological floor — gestational tissue lying free in vagina or specimen from operating room. 21 were acquired at time of therapeutic abortion (18-month period).	72	20	1	E–3
Hall & Källen (1964)	Not reported	Aborted placental tissue where no remnants of fetuses were found. Material is part of a collection for a systematic investigation of fetal wastage and malformation. Lund, Sweden, Department of Genetics and Department of Embryology.	Not reported	8	0	A–2

To estimate the incidence of trisomy 21 in terms of conceptions, let us assume that 15 per cent of conceptions terminate in a fetal death, 4 per cent of which have trisomy 21, and that 1.5 per 1,000 live-born have trisomy 21. The relationships which result would be as follows:

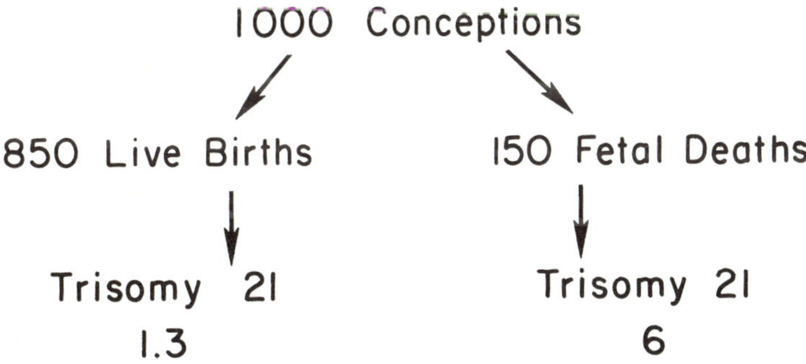

Thus, the incidence rate per 1,000 conceptions would be 7.3. In order to obtain a more acceptable estimate, one should adjust for maternal age and take into account the variations in the frequency of abortions by maternal age, for there is the possibility that the frequency of trisomy 21 among abortions may vary with maternal age. Unfortunately, there are no data available to do this adequately.

From this computation, one can estimate that about 80 per cent of conceptions with trisomy 21 terminate in abortions and about 20 per cent go on to be live-born. This implies that in epidemiological studies of mongol births we are merely studying the "top of the iceberg." The restriction of epidemiological studies to cases of mongolism exclusively, limits the potential inferences regarding etiological factors of trisomy 21. It is quite possible that factors causing trisomy 21 are confounded with other factors that cause the fetus with trisomy 21 to abort or to survive the fetal period.

It would appear profitable to pursue these chromosomal studies of abortions further and to integrate them with other epidemiological studies of mongolism. There are, of course, technical problems in such studies which have been recently discussed by Carr (1967) and participants at the Geneva Conference (WHO).

Racial and Ethnic Groups

Epidemiologists and geneticists are interested in determining whether there are differences in the frequency of disease in different racial and ethnic groups, since they may reflect differences in environment, living habits, or possibly the genetic composition of the groups. A lead to possible specific etiological factors may be forthcoming from such observations.

For many years, it was believed that mongolism occurred only in the white (i.e., Caucasian) race. However, through the years, reports of mongols from practically every racial group and country have appeared, indicating that mongolism does occur in all races and ethnic groups. Despite these reports, very little definitive information is available on actual incidence rates for the many racial groups.

For Negroes, there are 3 reports of incidence rates. Parker reported an incidence rate of 1.16 per 1,000 Negro births in the U.S., which is not significantly different from that of 1.03 per 1,000 Caucasian births. Kahn reported a rate of 1 per 1,000 African live births in South Africa; however, it is difficult to evaluate this rate in the absence of information on the method of case ascertainment. The third report is from Babbott and Ingalls who analyzed the cases of mongolism stated on Pennsylvania birth certificates in 1960 and found an incidence of 0.43 per 1,000 white and 0.12 per 1,000 Negro live births. In view of the high degree of underreporting of mongolism on birth certificates, the racial difference may merely reflect differences in degree of diagnosis and reporting; therefore, caution must be exercised in judging this comparison.

For the Egyptians, Hashem and Sakr reported an incidence of 1.25 per 1,000 total births from one sector of Cairo.

Of interest are the observations by Davies in Israel. He was able to study 100 per cent of the pregnant residents of western Jerusalem during 1964–66, including the outcome of their pregnancies. The migration of Jews to Israel from different areas during the past several years enabled Davies to determine the frequency of mongolism among the different migrant groups according to continents of origin (Table 2–4).

The higher rates among migrants from Africa (essentially North Africa) are of interest, as well as the fact that the rates for all of the groups are generally higher than those reported in other series (Table 2–1). The differences may reflect differences in the maternal age distribution of the live births, although the maternal ages for the Asian group are higher than those for the Africans. Granted these results are preliminary and the number of cases studied small, further study appears worth-while. It should be noted that Davies's results are in contrast to those of Halevi, who reported a rate of 1.21 per 1,000 in Israel in 1959–60 among Ashkenazim (European origin) in contrast to 0.94 for those of Middle East origin; these rates were based on a retrospective review of obstetric records which would underestimate the rate.

The most extensive data recently became available from an investigation conducted under the auspices of the World Health Organization. This study involving 16 countries was conducted in 24 centers to ascertain the incidence of congenital malformations among births (Stevenson, Johnston, *et al.*). Information was obtained on 421,781 pregnancies in these areas during the period 1961–64 covering at least 10,000 births in each center; included among the malformations was

Table 2–4. Incidence of Mongolism (per 1,000 Live Births) by Continent of Origin, Western Jerusalem, Israel, 1964–66

	Continent of origin					
	Asia	Africa	Europe or America	Israel (Jews)	Israel (Non-Jews)	Total
Number	13	16	5	18	1	53
Rate per 1,000 live births	3.0	3.7	2.2	2.9	2.3	3.0

Source: Davies, A. M. 1968. Personal communication.

mongolism. Table 2–5 presents the incidence rates, standardized for maternal age, for the individual centers. Many of the differences in the reported incidence rates may represent sampling fluctuation, since the rates in many centers are based on small numbers of cases. In evaluating these differences, it is also necessary to take into account the differences in diagnostic criteria and sensitivity in recognition of mongolism that most certainly exist in these centers. These factors make it impossible to determine whether these reported differences represent real differences in incidence in these populations. Nonetheless, they do indicate the need for more definitive studies in selected countries.

It is of special interest that no cases of mongolism were reported from Alexandria, from the 2 centers in India, or among the 4,141 births to Indian mothers in Kuala Lumpur, and that only one case was reported among 3,119 births to Indian mothers in Singapore. The

Table 2–5. Incidence Rates of Mongolism Standardized for Maternal Age for Selected Centers in Various Countries

Country	Total number single births	Number of mongols	Maternal age-standardized incidence rate per 1,000 total births
Melbourne, Australia—center *A*	7,844	8	0.93
Melbourne, Australia—center *B*	3,921	6	2.09
Sao Paulo, Brazil	14,421	11	0.86
Santiago, Chile	23,720	37	1.34
Bogota, Colombia	18,812	10	0.57
Medellin, Colombia	20,459	18	0.81
Czechoslovakia	20,074	27	2.02
Alexandria, Egypt	9,598	0	0.00
Hong Kong	9,872	1	0.17
Bombay, India	39,498	0	0.00
Calcutta, India	19,191	0	0.00
Kuala Lumpur, Malaysia	15,937	3	0.16
Singapore, Malaysia	39,683	17	0.37
Mexico City, Mexico—center *A*	24,700	46	1.97
Mexico City, Mexico—center *B*	14,083	22	1.72
Belfast, Northern Ireland	28,091	28	1.07
Panama City, Panama	15,852	17	1.44
Manila, Philippines	29,669	17	0.54
Cape Town, South Africa	3,051	0	0.00
Johannesburg, South Africa	11,176	8	0.83
Pretoria, South Africa	10,025	6	0.59
Madrid, Spain	19,714	39	1.75
Ljubljana, Yugoslavia	8.888	20	3.89
Zagreb, Yugoslavia	8,416	6	2.47
Total	416,695	347	0.83

Source: Stevenson, A. C., Johnston, H. A., Stewart, M. I. P., & Golding, D. R. 1966. "Congenital malformations: A report of a study of series of consecutive births in 24 centres." *Bull. WHO*, Suppl. 34, 9–127.

analysis of the total experience among Indian mothers in all of these areas indicates that only one mongol birth was reported among nearly 66,000 births. Although this low rate may reflect a low degree of sensitivity in the recognition of mongolism in these centers, it is difficult to believe that the 66 cases expected, if a rate of 1 per 1,000 births had prevailed, would have gone unnoticed. The authors of the report indicate that correspondence with several of the local organizers of the study suggested that specific difficulties in their respective centers may have been responsible for missed cases.

This set of data on incidence rates in these countries is of considerable value, for it suggests geographical areas where potentially fruitful and more definitive studies can be conducted. For example, it would appear worth-while to carry out chromosomal surveys of all newborn in the countries with high and low rates, such as Yugoslavia and India. If these rates are confirmed by more definitive studies, it would then be desirable to proceed with appropriate epidemiological studies to determine the possible reasons for the differences.

An aspect of the possible influence of race that has captured the interest of several investigators is the relative frequency of different chromosomal types of mongols. Starkman and Shaw summarized the literature on the frequency of translocation among Negro mongols and found that of 31 Negro mongols, 6, or 20 per cent, had translocations, which is higher than the approximate 3 per cent reported in Caucasian populations (Table 2–6). However, in their own study of the chromosomes of 20 Negro mongols from 3 large state institutions in Michigan, they found no translocations. It is possible that the re-

Table 2–6. Negro Mongols Found in Literature Survey

	Number of Negro mongols		
Investigator and year of report	Total	With trisomy 21	With translocation
Hayashi (1962)	3	2	1
Migeon, Kaufmann, & Young (1962)	1		1
Sherz (1962)	1		1
Dekaban, Bender, & Economos (1963)	6	6	
Mercer, Keller, & Lansdale (1963)	1	1	
Walker, Carr, *et al.* (1963)	2	1	1
Tompkins (1964)	2	2	
Wilton (1964)	6	6	
Migeon (1965)	1	1	
Weinstein, Rucknagel, & Shaw (1965)	8	6	2

Source: Starkman, M. N. & Shaw M. W. 1967. "Atypical acrocentric chromosomes in Negro and Caucasian mongols." *Amer. J. Hum. Genet.* 19: 162–73.

ports in the literature represent biased reporting. Investigators tend to report the unusual or less frequent types of chromosomal mongols, which would therefore result in a higher frequency of translocation mongols.

Among the Japanese, Tonomura, Oishi, Matsunaga, and Kurita reported finding 6 translocations among 127 mongols, about 5 per cent, which is not too different from that observed in Caucasian populations.

Most recently, Huang, Emanuel, Lo, Liao, and Hsu summarized the reports of studies on the frequency of different chromosomal types of mongols in different countries, including Caucasian, Japanese, and Chinese populations. Limiting his summary to those series which contained 20 or more cases, the results clearly fail to show any differences in frequencies (Table 2–7).

From this review of available data, it becomes quite evident that more definitive information on the incidence rates of mongols from the different racial and ethnic groups in the countries throughout the world would be useful, but must be obtained in as uniform and systematic a manner as is possible in order to be of value in the search for etiological factors.

Table 2–7. Percentage Frequencies of the Major Chromosomal Anomalies in Down's Syndrome

Country	Investigator and year of report	Number	Chromosomal anomalies: Trisomy G	D/G Translocation	G/G Translocation	Trisomy G/Normal mosaic
United States	Hayashi (1963)	78	93.59	3.85	0.00	2.56
Canada	Sergovich, Soltan, & Carr (1964)	96	97.92	0.00	2.08	0.00
United Kingdom	Chitham & MacIver (1965)	103	93.20	2.91	0.97	2.91
	Hamerton, Giannelli, & Polani (1965)	155	92.90	1.29	2.58	3.23
	Richards, Stewart, *et al.* (1965)	224	95.09	0.89	1.34	2.68
Sweden	Hall (1964)	58	98.28	1.72	0.00	0.00
	Gustavson (1964)	99	92.93	1.01	4.04	2.02
Finland	Aula & Hjelt (1964)	23	91.30	4.35	0.00	4.35
	Edgren, De La Chapelle, & Käariäien (1966)	72	98.61	0.00	0.00	1.39
Japan	Makino (1964)	95	98.95	1.05	0.00	0.00
Taiwan	Huang, Emanuel, *et al.* (1967)	77	94.81	2.60	1.30	1.30
Total	All studies	1,080	95.19	1.48	1.39	1.94

Source: Huang, S. W., Emanuel, I., Lo, J., Liao, S. K., & Hsu, C-C. 1967. "A cytogenetic study of 77 Chinese children with Down's syndrome." *J. Ment. Defic. Res.* 11: 147–52.

Maternal Age

One of the well-substantiated observations concerning mongolism is its increased incidence with advancing maternal age. Table 2–8 summarizes most of the studies which provide incidence rates for mongolism in the various maternal age groups, and Figure 2–1 presents the data in terms of logarithms of incidence rates. Despite differences in methods of ascertainment in these studies (Table 2–1), there is a notable consistency in the findings.

Some investigators have used a different approach to study the effect of maternal age, an indirect one; the maternal age distribution of a group of mongols is compared to a similar distribution of controls, or to a population of births, and a relative incidence by age group is computed by calculating the ratio of the per cent of mongols to the per cent of controls. The results of several of these studies are summarized in Table 2–9 and Figure 2–2. It is noteworthy that the shapes of the curves in Figures 2–1 and 2–2 are similar.

In general these data indicate that the risk of mongolism remains practically constant up to 30 years, after which it continues to increase during the remainder of the reproductive period; the curve of the logarithms of the rates from the 30 through 35 year age group onward is almost linear, although a slight decrease in the rate of increase appears after 45 years of age. It is also noteworthy that the same general pattern of the relationship between mongolism and maternal age persists during different time periods and in different countries.

Table 2–8. Summary of Selected Studies on Incidence Rates of Mongolism (per 1,000 Births) by Maternal Age, 1923–64

	Investigator, year of report, and years of study							
Maternal age	Øster (1956) 1923–44	Collmann & Stoller (1962) 1942–57	Carter & MacCarthy (1951) 1943–49	Stark & Mantel (1966) 1950–64	Renwick, Miller, & Patterson (1964) 1955	Halevi (1967) 1959–60	Stevenson, Johnston, *et al.* (1966) 1961–64	Davidenkova, Shtil'bans, *et al.* (1964) Not reported
<15	—	—	—	—	—	—	0.30	—
15–19	—	—	—	—	—	—	0.50	—
<20	0.61	0.43	0.00	0.43	0.36	0.37	—	0.17
20–24	0.69	0.62	0.28	0.43	0.36	0.45	0.32	0.48
25–29	0.70	0.83	0.29	0.51	0.43	0.46	0.38	0.46
30–34	1.14	1.15	1.72	0.87	0.61	1.07	1.63	0.80
35–39	3.58	3.50	3.52	2.64	1.89	2.74	2.11	2.66
40–44	10.30	9.93	14.18	—	7.80	7.53	6.34	9.60
40+	—	—	—	8.59	—	—	—	—
45+	17.80	22.00	26.32	—	11.44	3.19	16.65	9.61

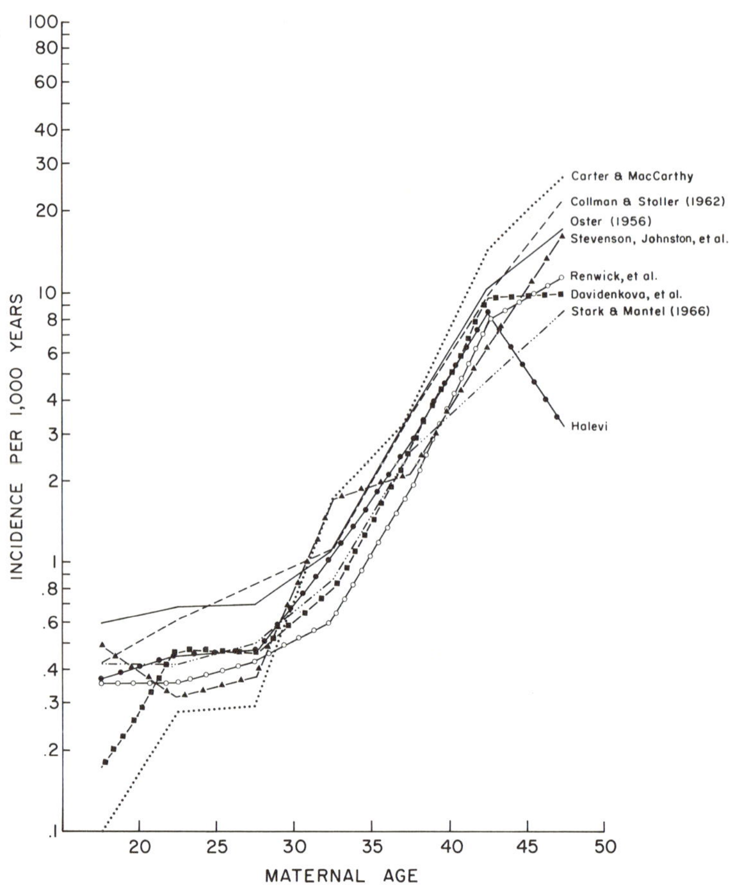

Figure 2–1. Incidence Rates of Mongolism by Maternal Age from Selected Studies, 1923–64.

In interpreting this relationship of mongolism with maternal age, it is necessary to determine if it is primary or a reflection in whole or in part, of a relationship with birth order or paternal age or both, since maternal age, paternal age, and birth order are all interrelated. It is of historical interest that one of the early observations was that mongols were frequently born last (Shuttleworth), leading clinicians to believe that mongolism was due to the exhaustion of maternal reproductive powers from frequent childbearing. The confounding influence of these 3 related factors made it essential to distinguish between their respective effects. Penrose (1939), in a series of papers in the 1930s, developed some statistical analytical methods which in-

Table 2–9. Summary of Selected Studies of Relative Frequency of Mongolism (per cent Mongols/per cent Controls) by Maternal Age

Maternal age	Matsunaga (1963)	Chitham & MacIver (1965)	Akesson & Forssman (1966) *A*	Akesson & Forssman (1966) *B*	Tonomura, Oishi, *et al.* (1966)
<20	0.46	0.44	0.33	0.30	—
15–24	—	—	—	—	0.42
20–24	0.53	0.56	0.40	0.33	—
25–29	0.52	0.55	0.39	0.44	0.88
30–34	0.85	0.62	0.69	0.72	1.38
35–39	2.48	2.30	1.85	2.26	3.35
40–44	5.31	6.01	5.73	7.20	—
40+	—	—	—	—	4.20
45+	18.73	10.71	10.32	16.71	—

Note: Akesson & Forssman (1966). *A* = Swedish patients, *B* = English patients.

dicated that maternal age was the principal variable and paternal age and order of birth had no effect. The methods used by Penrose were indirect ones, particularly the one differentiating between the effects of maternal and paternal age. More recently, Sigler, Lilienfeld, Cohen, and Westlake (1965*b*) used a more direct approach in evaluating the relative importance of maternal and paternal ages in a study in Baltimore. The results of their study will be described in more detail later. At this point in our discussion it is sufficient to mention that this analysis did not indicate any paternal age effect.

In analyzing the maternal age distributions of mongol children, several investigators have called attention to bimodality in the curve—that is, a smaller peak in the maternal age distribution for the younger and a larger peak for the older mothers of mongols (Figure 2–3). This observation, Penrose (1939) postulated to mean that there are essentially 2 components, one which he termed class *A*, age-independent, and the other class *B*, age-dependent. The latter curve essentially consists of an exponential increase of incidence with advancing maternal age. He went on to estimate the relative proportion of these 2 components by comparing the maternal age per cent distribution of mongol cases with that of total births in the population. Originally, Penrose had estimated that 22 per cent of the mongols were age-independent cases; however, in a more recent analysis of a series of maternal age distributions of cases collected in 11 countries, he estimated that 33 to 50 per cent are in the age-independent class *A*, the per cent varying with the maternal age distribution of the selected cases.

Before proceeding to consider the issue of 2 components, it would be well to consider the question of the bimodality of the age distribution. It has been pointed out by Sigler, Lilienfeld, Cohen, and Westlake (1965*b*) that this early peak in the age distribution may represent a statistical artifact, reflecting the relatively larger number of births between the ages of 20 and 29 in the general population. This can be demonstrated as follows: 2 theoretical populations of births have been developed and their maternal age distributions, similar to those found in actual populations, are shown in Table 2–10. In Population *A*, the peak in the maternal age distribution for total births has been placed in the 25 to 29 year age group, and in Population *B* in the 20 to 24 year age group. By applying the same age-specific incidence rates for Down's syndrome to each of these theoretical popula-

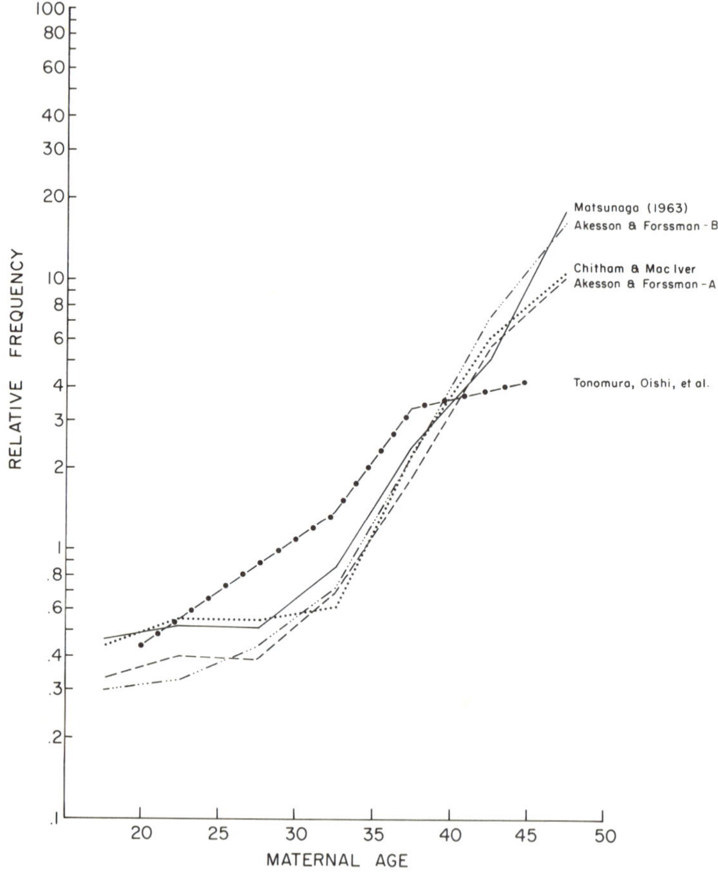

Figure 2–2. Relative Frequency of Mongolism (per cent Mongols /per cent Controls) by Maternal Age.

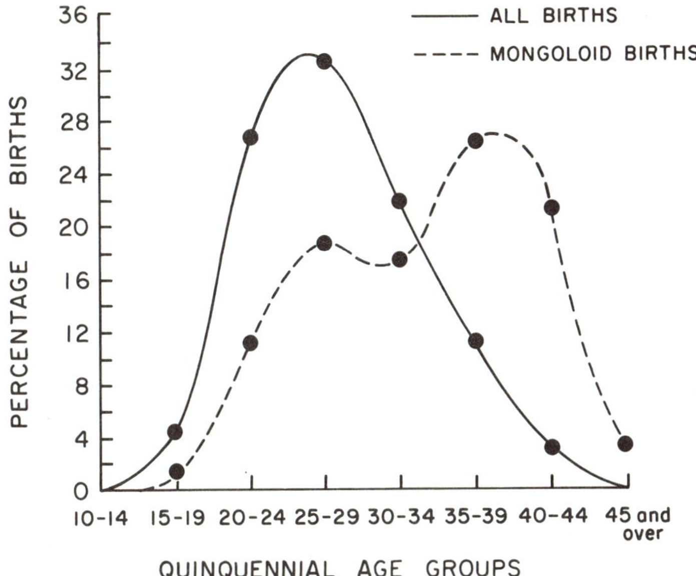

Figure 2–3. Distribution of All Births and Mongol Births by Maternal Age, Victoria, Australia 1942–57 (*from: Collmann & Stoller, 1962*).

tions, the expected number of cases for each maternal age group can be calculated. In each population, peaks are found in the maternal age distribution of mongolism which correspond exactly to the peaks in the theoretical populations of births. The effect of changing the peak of the birth distribution has been the movement of the secondary maternal age peak among mongols from age group 25 through 29 up to group 20 through 24 (Table 2–10 and Figure 2–4). In addition, it is clear from the age-specific incidence rates (Figure 2–1) that the risk of mongolism does not increase in the 20 to 29 year maternal age group.

Despite the possible interpretation of bimodality, it would be helpful to think in terms of separating mongols into 2 components based on maternal age-specific incidence rates. Examination of Figures 2–1 and 2–2, which present these data, indicates that prior to 35 years of age, the rate is relatively stable. If one assumes, as did Penrose, that the rate at the youngest age is almost entirely age-independent, a not too unreasonable assumption, one could subtract this rate from all subsequent rates and then determine the rates for age-dependent mongolism.

Table 2–10. Theoretical Maternal Age Distributions of 2 Populations, Demonstrating the Movement of the Early Down's Maternal Age Peak with Actual Age-Specific Incidence Rates Held Constant

Maternal age	Age-specific incidence per 1,000 births	Number of births in general populations (theoretical)		Number and per cent of cases of Down's syndrome expected: Population *A*		Population *B*	
		Population *A*	Population *B*	Number	Per cent	Number	Per cent
15–19	0.00	10,000	10,000	0	00.0	0	00.0
20–24	0.28	71,428	103,448	20	12.5	29	18.1
25–29	0.29	103,448	71,428	30	18.8	21	13.1
30–34	1.72	15,116	15,116	26	16.2	26	16.2
35–39	3.52	12,500	12,500	44	27.5	44	27.5
40–44	14.18	2,397	2,397	34	21.2	34	21.3
45+	26.32	227	227	6	3.8	6	3.8
Total	1.51	215,116	215,116	160	100	160	100

Note: These theoretical populations are similar in shape to actual populations and are similar to one another except for a reversal between the 20–24 and 25–29 age groups in regard to number of births. Age-specific incidence rates from Carter & MacCarthy (1951).

Source: Sigler, A. T., Lilienfeld, A. M., Cohen, B. H., & Westlake, J. E. 1965*b*. "Parental age in Down's syndrome (mongolism)." *J. Pediat.* 67: 631–42.

Computations of this type are presented in Table 2–11 using Øster's (1956) incidence rates. Thus, if one assumes a rate of 0.6 per 1,000 as the age-independent rate, this represents 9 per cent of the cases where maternal age is under 20 years. Subtraction of these rates from the total rates is presented in column 3 and the proportion of the total rate in each maternal age group that is age-independent is presented in column 4.

To estimate the actual proportion of cases in both of these groups from a realistic viewpoint, the maternal age distribution of live births in the U.S. was used to compute the expected number of total mongols, number of age-dependent and age-independent mongols using Øster's (1956) maternal age-specific incidence rates (Table 2–12). We note that with these incidence rates, we would expect a total of 5,220 mongols, of which about 50 per cent would be maternal age-independent.

It should be pointed out that the proportion of mongols that is estimated to be independent of maternal age will vary depending upon the maternal age distribution of live births. Thus, if all births were among mothers under 30 years of age, clearly a larger proportion would be maternal age-independent, and the converse would be true if a large proportion of births were among mothers over 40 years of age. It is important to remember the distinction when inter-

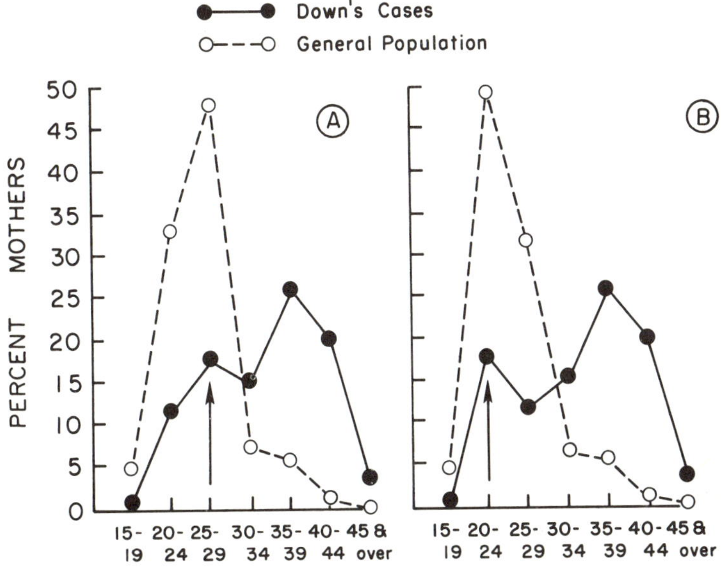

Figure 2–4. Theoretical Distributions of General Populations *A* and *B* with Corresponding Distributions of Cases of Down's Syndrome Using the Same Age-Specific Incidence Rates on Each Population (*from: Sigler, Lilienfeld, et al., 1965b*).

preting any data on the proportions of mongols that are age-dependent or age-independent.

One interesting aspect of the maternal age-mongolism relationship relates to the possible control of mongolism through family planning. Thus, it would be of interest to speculate on what proportion of mongol births would be prevented if reproduction ceased at specified ages. This is illustrated in Table 2–13 which presents the cumulative expected number and per cent of mongols starting at the older ages using the data on number of births and incidence rates of mongolism from Table 2–12. One finds that about 20 per cent of mongol births would be born to mothers 40 years of age and over. This suggests that a relatively simple means of decreasing the number of mongols is available by limiting the number of pregnancies among older mothers. One would expect a decrease of between 20 to 45 per cent in the frequency of mongolism if family limitation was practiced by mothers 35 to 40 years of age.

Cytological Types of Mongols and Maternal Age. There has been considerable interest in determining whether there is any differen-

Table 2–11. Estimation of the Proportion of Maternal Age-Independent and Age-Dependent Mongols

Maternal age	Incidence rates (per 1,000) Total (1)	Age-independent *A* (2)	Age-dependent *B* (3)	Proportion of age-independent mongols (4) = (2/1)
<20	0.61	0.6	0.01	0.98
20–24	0.69	0.6	0.09	0.87
25–29	0.70	0.6	0.10	0.86
30–34	1.14	0.6	0.54	0.53
35–39	3.58	0.6	2.98	0.17
40–44	10.30	0.6	9.70	0.06
45+	17.80	0.6	17.20	0.03

tial frequency in the different forms of mongolism by maternal age. Most recently Wright, Day, Muller, and Weinhouse summarized 19 reports on 1,302 patients (Tables 2–14 and 2–15). It is clear from Table 2–14 that translocations are more frequent at young maternal ages; 8.9 per cent of mongols born to mothers under 30 years of age are translocation mongols, as compared to 2.1 per cent over 30 years of age. Subdividing the translocations into the different types—sporadic and inherited—we note that at younger maternal ages, about 41 per cent of the D/G 21 translocations are inherited and 59 per cent are sporadic, i.e., the parents have normal chromosomal patterns. On the other hand, only 8 per cent of the G/G 21 translocations are inherited and 92 per cent are sporadic. Viewing the matter in terms of the frequency of sporadic translocation of both types by maternal age, we note that among the young mothers 75 per cent are sporadic as

Table 2–12. Estimation of the Expected Number of Total and Maternal Age-Independent and Age-Dependent Mongols

Maternal age	Live births U.S. 1960	Expected number of mongols *A* Total	*B* Age-independent	*C* Age-dependent
<20	593,746	362.1	356.2	5.9
20–24	1,426,912	984.5	856.1	128.4
25–29	1,092,816	765.0	655.7	109.3
30–34	687,722	784.0	412.6	371.4
35–39	359,908	1,288.4	215.9	1,072.5
40–44	91,564	943.1	54.9	888.2
45+	5,182	92.2	3.1	89.1

Note: Columns *A*, *B*, and *C* based on rates in column (1), (2), and (3) respectively, of Table 2–11.

Source: U.S. Department of Health, Education, and Welfare. 1962. Public Health Service. *Vital Statistics of the United States, 1960,* Vol. 1, Natality, U.S. Government Printing Office.

Table 2–13. The Cumulative Expected Number and Per Cent of Mongol Births (from Older to Younger Maternal Ages) by Maternal Age Estimated for U.S. Live Births, 1960

Maternal age	Cumulative expected number of mongols	
	Number	Per cent
<20	5,219	100.0
20–24	4,857	93.1
25–29	3,873	74.2
30–34	3,108	59.6
35–39	2,324	44.6
40–44	1,035	19.9
45+	92	1.8

compared to 85 per cent among the older mothers. These differences are not statistically significant and may be the result of the small number of cases in these groups.

Interpretation of the Maternal Age Effect. The increasing incidence of mongolism with increasing maternal age is probably the most striking epidemiological characteristic of mongolism. It reflects an increase in the frequency of nondisjunction with advancing maternal age, and several hypotheses have been offered to explain this phenomenon.

One hypothesis is that of uterine selection. This states that the frequency of nondisjunction is equal at all ages but that the "acceptability" for uterine implantation of the trisomic fertilized ovum varies with age, i.e., the uterus becoming less selective with increasing age. This would presuppose less of an interval between marriage and a first affected child, but not of a normal first-born among younger mothers. Matsunaga (1967*a*) presented some data that were consistent with this hypothesis, but they were not statistically significant (Table 2–16). Although this might not appear to be a biologically reasonable hypothesis, it should be tested further using new data from

Table 2–14. Chromosomal Findings on Patients with Down's Syndrome—Pooled Data from Several Studies

Maternal age	Number of patients	Trisomy 21 and mosaics	D/G21 translocation				G/G21 translocation				Translocations (per cent)
			Sporadic	Inherited	Unknown	Total	Sporadic	Inherited	Unknown	Total	
<30	722	658	16	11	6	33	23	2	6	31	8.9
30+	660	646	5	2	—	7	6	—	1	7	2.1
Total	1,382	1,304	21	13	6	40	29	2	7	38	

Source: Wright, S. W., Day, R. W., Muller, H., & Weinhouse, R. 1967. "The frequency of trisomy and translocation in Down's syndrome." *J. Pediat.* 70: 420–24.

Table 2–15. Frequencies and Proportions of Inherited and Sporadic Translocations

	D/G21 translocation		G/G21 translocation	
	Sporadic	Inherited	Sporadic	Inherited
Maternal age <30				
Number	16	11	23	2
Per cent	59	41	92	8
Sporadic translocations = 39/52 = 75 per cent				
Inherited translocations = 13/52 = 25 per cent				
Maternal age 30+				
Number	5	2	6	0
Per cent	71	29	100	0
Sporadic translocations = 11/13 = 84.6 per cent				
Inherited translocations = 2/13 = 15.4 per cent				

Note: Data from Table 2–14.
Source: Wright, S. W., Day, R. W., Muller, H., & Weinhouse, R. 1967. "The frequency of trisomy and translocation in Down's syndrome." *J. Pediat.* 70: 420–24.

other sources, particularly since it has been shown experimentally that fertilized ova transferred from young to old hamsters had a poorer survival rate than those implanted in young hamsters (Blaha). From this it was concluded that the uterine environment in older animals prevented normal nidation.

Laboratory experiments have also demonstrated that delayed fertilization of the mammalian ovum produces an increase in the frequency of abnormal and unsuccessful cleavages, structurally abnormal embryos, and embryonic resorption or abortions (Blandau; Fugo & Butcher). An increased frequency of chromosomal abnormalities has also appeared following delayed fertilization (Austin; Butcher & Fugo). It would seem reasonable therefore to assume that delayed fertilization might be of etiological importance in mongolism.

Table 2–16. Mean Interval between Marriage and First Birth for 96 Mothers of Children with Down's Syndrome, Grouped According to Whether the First-born Child Is Affected or Not

Maternal age at time of first birth	Status of first child	Number	Mean interval ± S.D. (years)
19–24	Affected	9	1.61 ± 0.78
	Normal	12	1.83 ± 0.89
25–29	Affected	34	1.59 ± 1.14
	Normal	15	1.97 ± 1.43
30–34	Affected	12	3.25 ± 2.49
	Normal	8	2.50 ± 2.00
35–41	Affected	5	3.20 ± 2.05
	Normal	1	2.5

Source: Matsunaga, E. 1967*a*. "General discussion," in: Ciba Foundation Study Group No. 25, *Mongolism* (Boston: Little Brown and Company).

Recently German postulated that the maternal age effect was a reflection of decreasing frequency of coitus with increasing duration of marriage, thereby decreasing the proportion of time during which spermatozoa are deposited in the uterus. In older women, therefore, oocytes will be fertilized after several hours, in contrast to an immediate fertilization of oocytes in younger women. He attempted to test this hypothesis by determining the duration of marriage of 201 mothers by age at birth of mongols. He compared the distribution of durations of marriage for those 35 years of age and over with that for mothers age 39 through 45 of all births at the New York Hospital. German noted a bimodal distribution of durations of marriage among the mothers of all births, with a prominent mode for women of short marriage durations which was not present among mothers of mongol births of the same age group.

Subsequent to the publication of this paper, Penrose and Berg reported on similar data for a group of 988 mongols and 1,146 controls, but found no differences in duration of marriage (Table 2–17). Cannings and Cannings, using an indirect approach with a statistical model, concluded that German's "hypothesis is not sufficient to explain the change in incidence of mongolism with maternal age." An analysis similar to that of German's was carried out on the material collected by Sigler, Lilienfeld, Cohen, and Westlake (1965*a*) in Baltimore, which has more adequate controls. The results were not consistent with German's hypothesis.

A third possible explanation has been proposed by Penrose (1965) and Penrose and Smith. Penrose points out that the incidence of mongolism increases with the power of age and suggests that the error in the ovum, leading to nondisjunction, depends upon a succession of

Table 2–17. Duration of Marriage in Years by Age of Mother at Birth of Child

Maternal age	Mongols			Controls			Difference of means	Standard error of difference
	Number	Mean duration	S.D.	Number	Mean duration	S.D.		
15–24	96	2.13	1.18	282	2.06	1.13	+0.07	±0.14
25–29	152	4.32	2.58	364	4.35	2.59	−0.03	±0.25
30–34	147	6.84	3.82	271	7.11	3.78	−0.27	±0.39
35–39	281	11.04	5.30	166	10.52	5.08	+0.52	±0.51
40–49	312	14.28	6.25	63	13.15	6.03	+1.13	±0.91
All	988	9.54	6.45	1,146	5.82	4.66	+3.72	±0.25

Source: Penrose, L. S. & Berg, J. M. 1968. "Mongolism and duration of marriage." *Nature* 218: 300.

independent accidents, either chemical or physical processes associated with age. After an accumulation of "accidents," the meiotic division becomes irregular due to degeneration of the spindle mechanism. He has determined that the relative incidence figures by maternal age agree with the estimated number of 17 or more "breaks" causing nondisjunction. This hypothesis essentially states that aging per se increases the frequency of errors in meiotic division, such as nondisjunction. If this is an aging effect, one would expect it to operate in other types of chromosomal abnormalities. It is of special interest that the frequency of Klinefelter's syndrome also increases with maternal age. In addition, Jacobs, Brunton, Court-Brown, Doll, and Goldstein and Hamerton, Taylor, Angell, and McGuire have reported an increased frequency of chromosomal abnormalities in leucocytes with advancing age and suggest that one of the effects of aging is a generalized lowering of mitotic efficiency leading to nondisjunction.

A fourth explanation, which is similar to the aging hypothesis, goes on to suggest that the increase with age reflects the cumulative effects of exposure to environmental agents during a lifetime. It differs from the general aging hypothesis in that the events producing the damage to the spindle mechanism are not "accidental" but due to environmental factors including viruses, radiation, chemicals, etc. Data on many of these environmental agents are presented and discussed in appropriate sections of this book.

Of course, if one is willing to speculate, it is just possible that both a general aging effect and environmental exposures interact to produce the same end-result, the maternal age effect.

Paternal Age

It has been stated in this review that several of the studies do not show any relationship between paternal age and mongolism. At this point we shall attempt to document this statement with the more recently published data.

Milham and Gittelsohn analyzed birth certificates in New York State for the period, 1950–62; their data, showing incidence rates by maternal and paternal ages, are presented in Table 2–18. Tonomura, Oishi, Matsunaga, and Kurita analyzed the paternal age distribution of 127 patients born in Japan during 1951–65 and adjusted for maternal age, using the maternal-paternal age distributions of live births in Japan for 1952–63 (Table 2–19). No paternal age effect is apparent in either of these studies. There are other investigators who have studied the paternal age distribution of a series of mongols and concur with the reported absence of a paternal age effect, including Beolchini, Bariatti, and Morganti; Stark; and Greenberg.

For their study, referred to earlier, Sigler, Lilienfeld, Cohen, and Westlake (1965*b*) selected 216 cases of mongols born in Baltimore and a control group of births matched for hospital of birth, sex, date of birth, and maternal age at time of birth and compared the paternal age distributions of the cases and the controls (Table 2–20). No significant differences were noted, although an interesting pattern did emerge in the younger maternal ages (under 35), the mongol group fathers were younger than the controls, whereas among the older mothers (35 and over), the case fathers were older than the controls. This finding was not statistically significant, but if any similar observations are made in the future it should be more thoroughly investigated.

The possible influence of paternal age was again proposed by Penrose in 1962, while summarizing the paternal and maternal ages of mongols with a 21/22 translocation. Penrose and Smith have recently

Table 2–18. Mongolism Cases by Parental Ages, Upstate New York, 1950–62

Paternal age	Maternal age							
	Total	15–19	20–24	25–29	30–34	35–39	40–44	45+
	Number of mongols							
15–19	7	6	1					
20–24	90	24	59	6	1			
25–29	142	6	47	69	15	4	1	
30–34	183		10	58	84	26	5	
35–39	214		4	8	54	124	21	3
40–44	199			2	12	87	92	6
45–49	91			1	3	25	56	6
50+	35		2		2	6	15	10
Not stated	20	3	5	3	7	2		
Total	981	39	128	147	178	274	190	25
	Cases per 10,000 births							
15–19	1.8	1.9	2.1					
20–24	2.0	2.0	2.4	2.5	5.6			
25–29	1.9	2.4	1.5	2.0	4.5	12.8	20.9	
30–34	2.9		1.5	2.0	3.5	10.1	28.6	
35–39	5.8		3.2	1.3	3.2	10.6	25.2	
40–44	12.7			1.5	2.9	12.3	33.4	127.9
45–49	18.0			2.6	2.9	13.0	38.1	45.8
50+	17.5				5.0	8.6	27.4	120.6
Total	3.9	2.0	1.7	1.9	3.4	11.2	32.6	89.4

Source: Milham, S., Jr. & Gittelsohn, A. M. 1965. "Parental age and malformations." *Hum. Biol.* 37: 13–22.

Table 2–19. Paternal Age Distribution and Relative Incidence, after Exclusion of Maternal Age Effect

Paternal age	Number of mongols: Observed	Number of mongols: Expected	Number observed minus expected	X^2	Relative incidence observed/expected
15–19	0	0.04	−0.51	0.06	0.887
20–24	4	4.47			
25–29	36	36.99	−0.99	0.03	0.973
30–34	50	47.27	+2.73	0.16	1.058
35–39	27	22.83	+4.17	0.76	1.183
40–44	5	9.74	−4.74	2.31	0.513
45–49	5	4.08	−0.66	0.08	0.883
50–54	0	1.16			
55–59	0	0.31			
60+	0	0.11			
Total	127	127.00		3.40	1.000
Mean age	32.39	32.60			
S.D.	5.62	6.01			

Source: Tonomura, A., Oishi, H., Matsunaga, E., & Kurita, T. 1966. "Down's syndrome: A cytogenetic and statistical survey of 127 Japanese patients." *Jap. J. Hum. Genet.* 11: 1–16.

reviewed and summarized the case reports for this particular translocation which suggests a paternal age effect. Since these are pooled case reports without any controls, evaluation of the data becomes very difficult. In addition, these case reports represent a highly select group which may have a bias toward older fathers. If the paternal age is present only in this group of translocation mongols, it will be extremely difficult to confirm these observations in a systematic survey, for this particular type of mongol only represents about 1 per cent of all mongols.

Table 2–20. Matched Pair Analysis of Paternal Age with Maternal Age Controlled (Paired *t* Test)

Maternal age	Down's paternal age minus control paternal age: Number of fathers	Mean difference	S.D.	*t*	*P* Value
15–19	6	0	2.8	0	*NS*
20–24	34	0	4.3	0	*NS*
25–29	30	−0.07	5.9	0.07	*NS*
30–34	46	−3.07	5.5	3.79	<0.001
35–39	62	+0.45	7.6	0.66	*NS*
40+	37	+1.1	6.4	1.05	*NS*
All cases	215	−0.34	6.3	0.79	*NS*

Source: Sigler, A. T., Lilienfeld, A. M., Cohen, B. H., & Westlake, J. E. 1965*b*. "Parental age in Down's syndrome (mongolism)." *J. Pediat.* 67: 631–42.

Mantel and Stark have recently stated that, for various statistical reasons, the question of a paternal age effect in mongolism has not yet been resolved. In light of this comment, a recent report by Matsunaga (1967*b*) is of interest. He presented data on 331 cases of mongols born in Japan during 1952–57, and used the paternal and maternal age distributions of all births in Japan to adjust for maternal age and year of birth in order to study the possible influence of paternal age (Table 2–21). It is clear that the mean paternal age for mongols did not differ significantly from that in the general population. However, the relative incidence appeared to increase slightly with advancing paternal age, but Matsunaga did not find the regressions of relative incidence on paternal age to be statistically significant.

The data presented in this review, collected from several recent studies, all adequately controlled in contrast to some of the earlier studies, also fail to show any marked paternal age effect. The inherent limitations of these studies cannot, however, rule out completely a small or perhaps a moderate effect of paternal age. To accomplish this successfully would require a large-scale study of several thousand mongols, particularly because it would be essential to do chromosomal analyses of the mongols to determine whether paternal age effects are present in specific types of mongols.

Table 2–21. Relative Incidence of Down's Syndrome According to Paternal Age, with Maternal Age Controlled

Paternal age at birth of mongols	Number		Number observed minus expected	X^2	Relative incidence observed/ expected
	Observed	Expected			
<25	14	21.2	−7.2	2.45	0.66
25–29	77	79.7	−2.7	0.09	0.97
30–34	75	71.5	+3.5	0.17	1.05
35–39	73	65.1	+7.9	0.97	1.12
40–44	47	56.3	−9.3	1.55	0.83
45–49	32	27.0	+5.0	0.94	1.19
50+	13	10.2	+2.8	0.75	1.27
Total	331	331.0	0	6.92	1.00
Mean age	35.3	34.7		d.f. = 6	
Variance	62.15	59.95		$P > 0.3$	

Source: Matsunaga, E. 1967*b*. "Parental age, livebirth order and pregnancy-free interval in Down's syndrome in Japan," in: Ciba Foundation Study Group No. 25, *Mongolism* (Boston: Little, Brown and Company).

Grandparents' Age

Several investigators have been interested in the grandmother's age at the time of the birth of a mongol's mother. The underlying reason is that the mother of a mongol may be a chromosomal mosaic influenced by her mother's age (the grandmother of the mongol) at the time of her birth. Greenberg collected information in 1958 on all mongol children born during 1953–57 in Essex County, England, and compared this with information obtained on a sample of children born during 1953–57. Using the combined data, he estimated the probabilities of having a mongol child for the various combinations of young and old mothers and young and old grandmothers. From a summary of his data (Table 2–22), we note that young mothers (under 35) appear to have twice the risk of having a mongol child if their mothers (grandmothers of the mongol child) were 35 years of age and over at the time of their birth.

Stark examined grandparents' age in a study of the families of 117 mongols and compared them with a group of families of control births selected from birth certificates matched by maternal age. The maternal and paternal grandparents of the mongols and control children had similar age distributions. He did not separately examine grandparents' age in relation to maternal age at birth of the mongols. In a recent report, Forssman and Akesson (1967) compared the grandmother's age at the time of birth of mothers for different maternal ages at birth for 1,282 mongols and found no differences (Table 2–23).

The latter 2 reports do not agree with that of Greenberg, although it is clear that Forssman and Akesson's results would be more acceptable if they had had a control group for comparison. Greenberg's observation is an interesting one and appears worthy of further study.

Table 2–22. Probability of a Mongol (per 1,000 Births) by Mother's Age at Birth of Mongol and Grandmother's Age at Birth of the Mother

Grandmother's age at mother's birth	Mother's age at birth of mongol	Probability of a mongol per 1,000 births (95 per cent confidence interval)
<35	<35	0.46 (0.42–0.50)
>35	<35	0.90 (0.71–1.10)
<35	>35	4.47 (3.13–5.82)
>35	>35	4.70 (2.40–7.00)

Source: Greenberg, R. C. 1963. "Two factors influencing the births of mongols to younger mothers." *Med. Off.* 109: 62–64.

Birth Order

Early workers in this field eliminated the probability of an independent relationship between birth order and mongolism. However, in response to chromosomal studies, there has been renewed interest in the possible relationship of mongolism and birth order, and several studies have recently been published.

Beolchini, Bariatti, and Morganti compared a group of 421 mongols, born in Milan during 1940–60, with a randomly selected sample of 2,801 births. For each maternal age group he compared the mongol cases and controls with respect to birth order and found no significant difference. Stark and Mantel (1966) did a similar study for 2,432 mongol children born in southern Michigan during 1950–64. They obtained the maternal age and birth order distribution of all live births in this area and computed specific rates (Table 2–24). It seems quite clear that there is no birth order effect that is independent of a maternal age effect.

In contrast are the findings of Smith and Record (1955*a*) and Tonomura, Oishi, Matsunaga, and Kurita, who found an excess frequency of first-order births among mongols, although the latter points out the possibility of a bias in the selection of the children they studied (Table 2–25). For example, it is possible that large teaching centers and hospitals may attract first-born mongols more often than those of higher birth orders, and, of course, birth control may have an effect; after having a first-born mongol, a mother may decide not to

Table 2–23. Maternal Age at Birth of 1,282 Patients with Down's Syndrome, by Grandmaternal Age at Birth of Mothers

Grand-maternal age	Maternal age						
	<20	20–24	25–29	30–34	35–39	40–44	45+
<20	2	4	6	2	1	7	1
20–24	4	21	26	32	48	66	16
25–29	8	32	38	45	92	101	21
30–34	6	22	40	50	77	104	22
35–39		17	23	33	68	78	12
40–44		14	19	19	27	50	13
45+		1	1		5	4	4
Total	20	111	153	181	318	410	89
Mean		30.2		31.0		31.3	
S.D.		6.7		6.3		6.7	

Source: Forssman, H. & Akesson, H. O. 1967. "Consanguineous marriages and mongolism," in: Ciba Foundation Study Group No. 25, *Mongolism* (Boston: Little, Brown and Company).

Table 2–24. Mongolism Occurrence Rates per 1,000 Live Births by Age of Mother and Birth Order, Lower Michigan, 1950–64

Maternal age	Birth order					Total	
	1	2	3	4	5+	Crude	Adjusted
<20	46.9	36.0	(20.7)	(45.3)	(00.0)	43.2	31.3
20–24	42.6	47.1	40.2	39.3	23.7	42.8	39.9
25–29	53.3	51.3	51.7	48.6	51.3	51.2	51.6
30–34	102.6	101.1	84.1	87.7	75.5	86.6	92.4
35–39	270.5	299.2	242.2	242.2	246.5	263.8	272.1
40+	850.9	753.6	864.6	940.1	851.7	858.9	839.9
Total							
Crude	56.7	68.5	81.4	114.4	165.6	89.1	
Adjusted	93.2	92.9	83.7	92.4	74.4		

Note: Rates in parentheses are based on fewer than 10 cases.
Source: Stark, C. R. & Mantel, N. 1966. "Effects of maternal age and birth order on the risk of mongolism and leukemia." *J. Nat. Cancer Inst.* 37: 687–98.

have any additional children. This is suggested by the results of a study by Matsunaga (1967*b*) where he analyzed the birth order distribution of a series of mongols in Japan by determining the expected number of cases in each birth order from the vital statistics data on all live births and found a higher observed-expected ratio for mongols; but he also found a similar pattern for other types of mental defectives (Table 2–26).

It is clear that most of the studies do not show a birth order effect, but some do suggest a higher risk for first-order births after maternal age is taken into account. This may reflect a biased selection of cases, or possibly the effects of the practice of birth control. However, before completely dismissing any possible effect of birth order, which ad-

Table 2–25. Distribution of Live-Birth Rank, after Exclusion of Maternal Age Effect

Live-birth rank	Number		Number observed minus expected	X^2
	Observed	Expected		
1	71	42.24	+28.76	19.58
2	35	42.37	−7.37	1.28
3	15	20.80	−5.80	1.62
4	4	9.33	−15.59	10.84
5+	2	12.26		
Total	127	127.00	0	33.32 (d.f. = 3, $P < 0.001$)

Source: Tonomura, A., Oishi, H., Matsunaga, E., & Kurita, T. 1966. "Down's syndrome: A cytogenetic and statistical survey of 127 Japanese patients." *Jap. J. Hum. Genet* 11: 1–16.

mittedly would be a small one at best, more carefully planned, large-scale population studies would be in order.

One of the difficulties in studying the influence of birth order in mongolism is that the birth order may in fact be influenced by the effect of the birth of the mongol on the mother's reproductive performance. To adequately study the effect of birth order, it would be necessary to compare the birth order distributions of mongols and controls for each maternal age group, as well as for family size. This would take into account both possible confounding effects, maternal age, and the effect of reproductive performance. It would be of interest to thoroughly clarify the effect of birth order, although the present impression is that its effect, if any, must be a modest one.

Table 2–26. Relative Incidence of Down's Syndrome and Other Mental Defects for Each Rank in the Live-Birth Order, with Maternal Age Controlled

Down's syndrome							
	Number of cases from institutions						
Ranks in live-birth order	Category *A*			Categories *B* and *C*			All cases
	Observed	Expected	Observed/ Expected	Observed	Expected	Observed/ Expected	Observed/ Expected
1	116	93.5	1.24	85	59.5	1.43	1.31
2	122	86.1	1.42	76	57.6	1.32	1.38
3	83	72.6	1.14	62	50.2	1.24	1.18
4	55	61.7	0.89	34	39.7	0.86	0.88
5	50	52.6	0.95	29	29.8	0.97	0.96
6	32	45.5	0.70	10	23.7	0.42	0.61
7+	62	108.0	0.57	18	53.6	0.34	0.50
Total	520	520.0	1.00	314	314.1	1.00	1.00

Mental defects other than Down's syndrome							
	Number of cases from institutions						
Ranks in live-birth order	Category *A*			Categories *B* and *C*			All cases
	Observed	Expected	Observed/ Expected	Observed	Expected	Observed/ Expected	Observed/ Expected
1	148	115.9	1.28	97	81.0	1.20	1.24
2	128	105.3	1.22	81	71.4	1.13	1.18
3	74	80.3	0.92	56	50.6	1.11	0.99
4	50	53.5	0.94	16	28.7	0.56	0.80
5	20	33.7	0.59	7	15.2	0.40	0.55
6	16	21.9	0.73	7	8.5	0.82	0.76
7+	13	38.3	0.34	5	13.6	0.37	0.35
Total	449	448.9	1.00	269	269.0	1.00	1.00

Source: Matsunaga, E. 1967*b*. "Parental age, live-birth order and pregnancy-free interval in Down's syndrome in Japan," in: Ciba Foundation Study Group No. 25, *Mongolism* (Boston: Little, Brown and Company).

3:

Distribution in Time and Space

Clustering

One distinguishing characteristic of the distribution of a disease in a population is the occurrence of the disease in "clusters," i.e., the aggregation of cases of the disease close together in space and/or time. The term "clustering" can be used broadly to define aggregation in space alone, time alone, or in both time and space. If used in a very broad sense, practically every epidemiological aspect of a disease can be considered in terms of clusters. For example, if there is a difference in incidence rates in different countries or in different geographical areas, such as urban-rural areas, this can be considered clustering in space; familial aggregation similarly may be regarded as a form of clustering. Temporal clustering can be sufficiently encompassing to include trends of incidence rates over time, as well as seasonal fluctuation.

Each different form of clustering leads to the development of different etiological hypotheses, and sudden changes in time may be suggestive of temporal changes in exposure to environmental factors. Clustering of cases in both time and space may suggest that a communicable, possibly infectious agent, is operative while seasonal variation may also suggest infectious agents. The demonstration of certain types of clusters can be relatively straightforward, whereas others may be more subtle and more difficult to isolate or differentiate. The concentration of disease in a specific locality may be revealed by an increased incidence rate and temporal variation by changes in incidence rates over time. A low order of temporo-spatial clustering poses many statistical problems which have been recently reviewed by Mantel, who presents some rather detailed statistical tests for evaluating the occurrence of disease clusters.

In the literature on mongolism, the term "clusters" has been applied broadly, i.e., including temporal alone, spatial alone, and temporo-spatial clustering. We would prefer a more restricted use of the term "clusters" to indicate temporo-spatial clustering and to use terms such as temporal trends, seasonal trends, etc., for the more explicit type of observations. We will try to differentiate between these different types although there will always be some overlapping.

Table 3–1 summarizes 11 studies on the temporo-spatial clustering of mongolism. Many of these studies pose methodological problems and most of them consist of retrospective analyses of cases reported from a variety of sources. No doubt there has been variability in the criteria used in the diagnosis of mongolism and also in the ascertainment of cases; from this viewpoint these studies are not comparable. In addition the results are not consistent with each other and in some instances it is not even clear whether the results are statistically significant. Recently several of these studies were reviewed by Day.

The first report suggesting temporo-spatial clustering was by Pleydell. Upon noticing that mongol children in Northamptonshire, England, appeared to be born in groups, he ascertained from all possible sources all cases of mongolism born during 1944–55, as well as other congenital malformations, including congenital heart disease, harelip, and cleft palate. He judged that about two-thirds of the mongol births had occurred in small groups, with the remainder occurring sporadically. Pleydell noted no differences in frequency in urban and rural areas but did indicate that the "clusters" were present in the rural areas. The absence of a statistical analysis makes it difficult to determine whether any statistical significance can be ascribed to his observations. However, he does speculate on the possible role of streptococcal infections during pregnancy in the etiology of mongolism.

Collmann and Stoller (1962), as part of an epidemiological survey of mental deficiency in Victoria, Australia, compiled a register of mongols born during 1942–57, using every available source, and analyzed the trend of incidence rates and seasonal and geographical distributions. They reported the occurrence of a 5- to 6-year peri-

Table 3–1. Summary of Studies on Temporo-Spatial Clustering of Mongolism in Different Geographical Areas

Investigator and year of report	Time period	Geographical area	Method of study	Incidence of mongols per 1,000 births	Results
Lander, Forssman, & Akesson (1964)	1911–58	Sweden	Survey of all institutions for the mentally deficient in Sweden.	Not reported	Fewer cases of mongols born in September.
Collmann & Stoller (1962)	1942–57	Victoria, Australia	Retrospective evaluation of maternal age-adjusted incidence rates.	1.45	Inferred clustering in time and space and suggested relationship with disease. No seasonal variation.
Pleydell (1957)	1944–45	Northamptonshire, England	Retrospective evaluation of clusters of cases in time and space: no statistical analysis.	1.63	Inferred clustering in time and space and suggested relationship to streptococcal infection.
Stark & Mantel (1967)	1950–64	Michigan, U.S.	Statistical analysis of annual and seasonal incidence.	0.89	Unable to demonstrate clustering by years, seasons or months within seasons.
Leck (1966)	1950–65	Birmingham, England	Retrospective statistical analysis of residence of births by determining the space and time distribution of pairing of mongol births.	1.62	If non-random clustering occurs, it is of low intensity and contributes little to total incidence. Incidence lower in July December.
Greenberg (1963)	1953–57	Essex County, England	Not reported.	1.19	No seasonal variation for mothers over 35 years of age. For those under 35 years, higher frequency in May, August, and October.
Lunn (1959)	1953–58	Glasgow, Scotland	Survey to find every mongol child born in city area of Glasgow.	1.02	Geographical grouping of homes of mongols on city map showed no significant grouping —no seasonal variation.

Table 3–1. Continued

Investigator and year of report	Time period	Geographical area	Method of study	Incidence of mongols per 1,000 births	Results
Slater, Watson, & McDonald (1964)	1954–60	England and Wales	Survey of members and associates of College of General Practitioners of United Kingdom and Eire regarding congenital defects. Letters sent to 4,000 practitioners and 1,373 replied.	Not reported	No seasonal variation.
Heinrichs, Allan, & Nelson (1963)	1954–63	South Dakota, U.S.	Review of hospital records supplemented by interrogations and questionnaires.	2.88	Secular variation every 3½ to 4 years.
Halevi (1967)	1959–60	Israel	Reports of all congenital malformations from maternity departments. Records were also reviewed.	1.01	Higher frequency in October–December.
Robinson & Puck (1967)	1962–66	Denver, U.S.	Chromosome analysis in newborns in whom mongol diagnosis was suspected in 2 hospitals in Denver.	1.12	Small tendency for clustering of cases during April–October (not significant).

odicity for the cities in Victoria. A similar pattern was observed for the rural areas, although the peaks in the rural areas lagged one year behind those in the urban areas (Figure 3–1). They also reported a higher incidence in the urban than in the rural areas. Defining a "cluster" as a "group of from two to twenty-five mongols, the cases in each group having been born in a restricted area . . . and within twelve months of each other," they found that clusters accounted for 40 per cent of the mongol births. The authors interpreted these findings as suggestive of an etiological influence of an infective agent, probably infectious hepatitis. The survey was then extended to include the period 1958–62 and the same pattern was again noted. Stoller and Collmann (1965*a*; 1965*b*; 1965*c*) then matched the periodic occurrence of mongolism with the annual incidence of reported infectious diseases during 1952–64 and found that for infectious hepatitis, the incidence showed concordance with a 9-month lag. The 9-month lag was accepted since these investigators postulated that the virus infected the ovum prior to or about the time of conception (Figure 3–2).

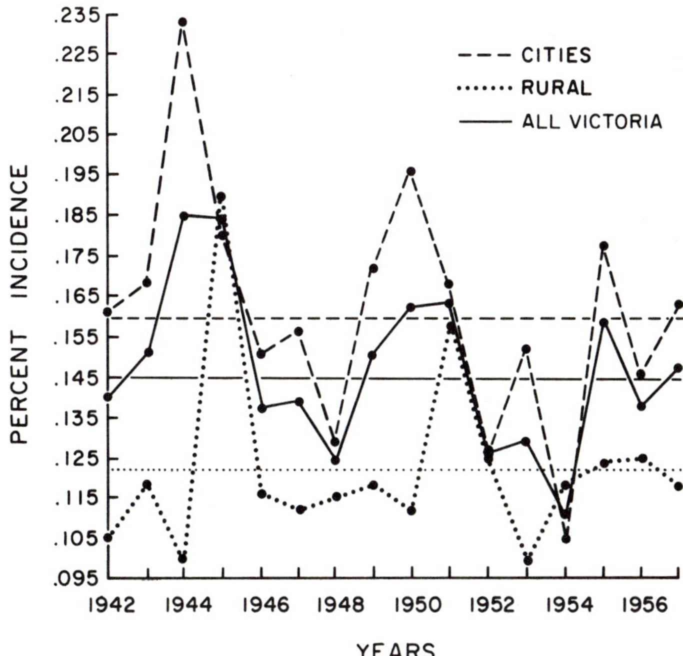

Figure 3–1. Annual Incidence of Mongol Births Adjusted for Annual Variations in the Quinquennial Age Distribution of All Parturient Mothers in the General Population, Victoria, Australia, 1942–57 (*from: Collmann & Stoller, 1962*).

Stoller and Collmann (1966) then attempted a more detailed analysis by dividing metropolitan Melbourne into 2 sections, a western and an eastern part; the western section was more densely populated than the eastern and more clusters of mongol births were observed in the east than in the west. They then determined the annual incidence of infectious hepatitis and mongolism in these 2 sections; these are presented in Table 3–2. The eastern section had a higher incidence of both infectious hepatitis and mongolism than the west, although the differences were statistically significant only for infectious hepatitis for each year but not for mongolism. In addition, they noted that the large increase of infectious hepatitis in the eastern part for 1956 was followed the next year by a high incidence of mongolism. However, it should be pointed out that this pattern was not present in the western part of the city (Table 3–2). The authors suggest that the higher incidence of mongolism in the eastern section may have been due to the inadequate sanitary facilities of this newly developed area, which was therefore more vulnerable to infectious hepatitis.

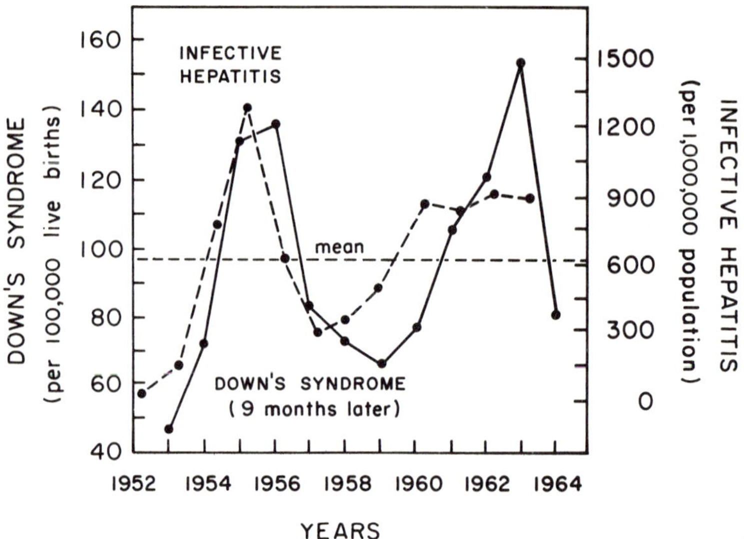

Figure 3–2. Annual Incidence of Infective Hepatitis (per Million) Followed 9 Months Later by Births (per 100,000 Live Births) of Children with Down's Syndrome, Victoria, Australia, 1952–64 (*from: Stoller & Collmann, 1965a*).

Collmann and Stoller's findings stimulated other investigators to confirm their results in other geographical areas. In 1963, Heinrichs, Allen, and Nelson reported that a retrospective review of hospital records showed 2 temporal clusters of mongol births during the period 1954–60 in South Dakota. Their data are presented in Table 3–3, together with computed annual incidence rates, as well as the incidence rate for the total time period. Using the incidence rate for the total period, expected numbers of mongols were computed for each year; the last column of the table indicates whether the observed numbers are greater than, less than or equal to the expected. In addition, 95 per cent confidence limits for the total incidence rate were computed; these are 1.77–4.47. This crude analysis does demonstrate the difficulty in inferring more than a random distribution from these data. However, this may simply be a reflection of the small number of cases. It is also noteworthy that the total incidence rate of mongolism is quite high, which may reflect an older maternal age distribution of total births.

Leck also conducted a retrospective survey in Birmingham, England for the period 1950–65, using data collected during a continuing study of malformations among children; the cases were ascertained by

Table 3–2. Numbers of Cases and Incidences of Infectious Hepatitis (per 100,000 of Population) and of Births of Children 9 Months Later with Down's Syndrome (per 100,000 Live Births) for the Eastern and Western Areas of Melbourne, Australia

	Infectious hepatitis					Down's syndrome			
	East		West			East		West	
Year	Number	Incidence	Number	Incidence	Year	Number	Incidence	Number	Incidence
1953–54	80	20.7	131	12.2	1954	11	119.3	24	110.1
1954–55	472	114.4	698	61.7	1955	17	172.2	36	159.8
1955–56	919	210.0	1,272	109.9	1956	30	285.1	26	115.1
1956–57	337	72.0	693	58.7	1957	21	185.5	33	137.1
Total	1,808	106.1	2,794	61.5	Total	79	193.0	119	130.8

Source: Stoller, A. & Collmann, R. D. 1966. "Area relationship between incidences of infectious hepatitis and of the births of children with Down's syndrome nine months later." *J. Ment. Defic. Res.* 10: 84–88.

a survey of all medical sources. He first compared, as did Collmann and Stoller, the annual trends of reported infectious hepatitis cases with those of mongolism; no relationship was found. He then analyzed the temporo-spatial distribution of cases of mongolism using a statistical method developed by Knox (1963). The authors' tabulation of the distribution of differences in time between all possible pairs of mongol births and in distance between residences is presented in Table 3–4 for two time periods 1950–54 and 1955–64. Leck interpreted these data as indicating that "if non-random clustering occurs, it is of low intensity and contributes little to total incidence." His general

Table 3–3. Annual Incidence Rate (per 1,000 Births) for Mongols and Expected Numbers Based on Total Rate for Births, South Dakota, 1954–61

Year	Number: Deliveries	Number: Mongols	Incidence rate per 1,000 (observed)	Expected number of mongols based on total rate	Observed minus expected rates
1954	817	1	1.22	2.36	−
1955	817	4	4.90	2.36	+
1956	832	2	2.40	2.40	=
1957	847	1	1.18	2.45	−
1958	727	3	4.13	2.10	+
1959	768	3	3.91	2.22	+
1960	691	2	2.89	2.00	=
1961	711	1	1.41	2.05	−
1962	617	2	3.24	1.78	=
1963 (First 2 months)	102	1	9.80	0.29	=
Total	6,929	20	2.89	−	

Source: Adapted from Heinrichs, E. H., Allen, S. W., & Nelson, P. S. 1963. "Simultaneous 18-trisomy and 21-trisomy cluster." *Lancet* 2: 468.

comment on Pleydell and Collmann and Stoller's results was, "The suggestion of these authors that Down's Syndrome is caused by an infection may be correct in some cases; but it seems likely that the etiological importance of this type of influence has been exaggerated."

These reports were followed by one by Stark and Fraumeni in which a comparison was made between the annual incidence rates of infectious hepatitis and mongolism in Michigan for the period, 1952–64; Collmann and Stoller's observations were not confirmed. Ceccarelli and Torbidoni also did a similar analysis in Italy for the period 1959–65, and they too were unable to confirm Collmann and Stoller's observations. Finally, Kogon, Kronmal, and Peterson did not succeed in confirming these relationships in Seattle and King County, Washington, U.S., for the period 1952–64. They also subjected Collmann and Stoller's data on clustering to a detailed statistical analysis using Monte Carlo methods and showed that the frequency of clusters reported could arise by chance alone.

However, Collmann and Stoller's observations did stimulate some experimental studies. Mella and Lang studied the effect of infectious hepatitis on the chromosomes of cells in peripheral blood by directly observing the leukocytes of patients with infectious hepatitis and also indirectly by adding the serum obtained from patients with infectious hepatitis to leukocyte cultures of healthy individuals. The chromosomes of leukocytes of patients with hepatitis had an increased inci-

Table 3–4. Proportion of Pairs of Cases of Mongolism Not More Than 4 Kilometers Apart, 1950–54 and 1955–64

	Years of mongols births					
	1950–54			1955–64		
Time apart (days)	Total number	Number 0–4 km. apart	Per cent 0–4 km. apart	Total number	Number 0–4 km. apart	Per cent 0–4 km. apart
0–50	650	207	31.8	1,531	408	26.6
51–100	579	161	27.8	1,480	329	22.2
101–150	486	139	28.6	1,468	373	25.4
151–200	483	136	28.2	1,503	342	22.8
201–250	528	179	33.9	1,445	366	25.3
251–300	497	166	33.4	1,404	329	23.4
301–350	515	156	30.3	1,386	325	23.4
351–400	523	129	24.7	1,373	316	23.0
Over 400	6,617	1,953	29.5	44,021	10,456	23.8
All pairs	10,878	3,226	29.7	55,611	13,244	23.8

Source: Leck, I. 1966. "Incidence and epidemicity of Down's syndrome." *Lancet* 2: 457–60.

dence of breaks, stickiness, abnormal numbers, deletions, and additions that had not been previously present. They also found that the serum of infectious hepatitis patients repeatedly inhibited leukocytic mitosis in culture. These findings are not totally unexpected since they have also been found in rubella. Of special interest is the report that mothers of mongol children have higher levels of thyroid antibodies than mothers of normal children and that patients with infectious hepatitis have an increase in thyroid antibodies (Dallaire & Kings-mill Flynn, 1967*a*).

The most recent analysis of temporo-spatial distribution was reported by Stark and Mantel (1967). They ascertained from a variety of medical sources that 2,431 mongol children were born during 1950–64 in the counties of the lower peninsula of Michigan. Their study reported the frequency distribution of mongol births in the counties as well as the annual and seasonal incidence rates (Table 3–5). Using relatively detailed and refined statistical methods, they too analyzed the temporo-spatial distribution; however, they were unable "to demonstrate any important aggregations of Down's Syndrome within the state of Michigan."

Table 3–5. Annual and Over-all Monthly Incidence of Down's Syndrome (per 100,000 Live Births) for the Lower Peninsula of Michigan, 1950–64

	Annual data				Monthly data, 15 years combined		
Year	Number of Down's syndrome births	Number of live births	Down's syndrome births per 100,000 live births	Month	Number of Down's syndrome births	Number of live births	Down's syndrome births per 100,000 live births
1950	136	154,261	88.2	January	178	219,584	81.1
1951	113	166,590	67.8	February	184	208,524	88.2
1952	151	171,628	88.0	March	212	229,020	92,6
1953	147	175,946	84.7	April	202	215,966	93.5
1954	150	185,094	81.0	May	187	227,511	82.2
1955	180	189,585	94.9	June	229	225,425	101.6
1956	202	199,184	101.4	July	228	239,100	95.4
1957	213	201,654	105.6	August	207	240,956	85.9
1958	186	195,756	95.0	September	205	237,912	86.2
1959	184	191,566	96.1	October	186	234,073	79.5
1960	164	188,342	87.1	November	215	219,812	97.8
1961	187	185,944	100.6	December	198	224,891	88.0
1962	177	175,772	100.7				
1963	134	172,202	77.8				
1964	105	169,250	62.0				
Total	2,431	2,722,774	89.3		2.431	2;722,774	89.3

Source: Stark, C. R. & Mantel, N. 1967. "Lack of seasonal or temporal-spatial clustering of Down's syndrome births in Michigan." *Amer. J. Epid.* 86: 199–213.

In evaluating Stark and Mantel's negative findings, one should note that they reported an incidence of mongolism of 0.89 per 1,000 births. This appears to be rather low and it is possible that there may have been incomplete ascertainment of cases with possible selective biases. This could create the appearance of no clustering, while clustering may actually be present.

In their discussion, Stark and Mantel raise several issues with regard to Collmann and Stoller's analysis. Their comments are worth quoting:

> Using a similar approach to interpret the data of Stoller and Collmann, we see several points which should be considered. The variety of notifiable infectious diseases to which Stoller and Collmann initially attempted to relate Down's syndrome, as well as the variety of statistical manipulations to which they subjected their data would readily have resulted in some formally significant results on the basis of chance alone. We note, also, that the 1953–64 data of Stoller and Collmann show a range of 6 to 20 cases of Down's syndrome per year, with an average of 12.7 per year. This range is consistent with simple Poisson variation. Further, the bulk of the hepatitis-Down's syndrome correlation reported by Stoller and Collmann appears to derive from the sharp rise in the 1952–55 portion of the hepatitis curve, a rise which could be related to the 1952 initiation of infectious hepatitis reporting in Australia.

Seasonal Distribution

Investigators for a long time have been interested in a possible correlation between all congenital malformations and season of birth, since many teratogenic factors do have a seasonal pattern. The reports of studies on congenital malformations other than mongolism have recently been reviewed by Bailar and Gurian, who commented on the many important questions that remain unanswered in this area.

In most of the reports on clusters reviewed in this chapter, the investigators have also reported on the seasonal distribution of mongol births, with varying results. Collmann and Stoller, and Stark and Mantel found none. Leck observed a lower incidence of mongols in July through December, but explained this as the result of underascertainment among undiagnosed children who died in infancy.

There have been several additional reports on the seasonal distribution of mongolism which are included in the summary in Table 3–1. Slater, Watson, and McDonald conducted a survey on congenital malformations among the members and associates of the College of General Practitioners of England and Ireland; of 4,000 practitioners, 1,373 replied. They found no seasonal variation; however, the low response rate in the survey may have resulted in a bias. On the other hand, Halevi, in his study of congenital malformations in Israel, reported a higher frequency of mongol births in the winter, October–December.

Lander, Forssman, and Akesson studied 1,192 mongol children, born in Sweden during 1911 to 1958, who were residents in institutions for the mentally retarded. They compared the month of birth of the cases with a weighted series of births in Sweden for the same time period and found significantly fewer births of mongol children in September. This report is of particular interest because it contains a rather complete discussion of the various nonbiological factors that can influence the seasonal distribution of births. In weighing these factors, they conclude that "it was probably impossible to get a satisfactory control series from official statistics and that one should thus regard any report that a certain group differed from the normal in season of birth with skepticism."

Greenberg studied a group of 148 mongols born during 1953–57 in a county in England. For the total group of mongol births and for the subgroup consisting of those born of mothers over 35 years of age no seasonal variation was observed. However, for those under 35 years of age, he noted a deficiency of mongol births in the first 4 months of the year and an excess in May, August, and October. His analysis suggested a possible relationship between the incidence of mongols and low temperatures, 7 to 8 calendar months before birth (Table 3–6). He hypothesized that atmospheric temperature would alter the distribution of body fluids and increase the viscosity of the protoplasm and "stickiness" of the chromosomes, which would influence the frequency of nondisjunction. This is an attractive hypothesis, but it is based on a small number of cases and, if true, one would expect greater differences in frequency of mongol births in different geographical areas than appear to be present.

An interesting study was conducted by Robinson and Puck in 2 hospitals in Denver during 1962–66. Virtually every baby born in these hospitals was examined for the possible presence of mongolism and chromosomal analysis was performed on every newborn with a suspect diagnosis. There was a slight suggestion of possible clustering

Table 3–6. Relationship between Monthly Temperature 8 Months before Birth and Frequency of Mongol Births

Average monthly temperature 8 calendar months before birth	Number		Excess over expectation
	Mongols born	Mongols expected	
Under 40° F.	16	9.0	+7.0
Over 40° and under 45°F.	13	10.3	+2.7
Over 45° and under 60°F.	31	34.9	−3.9
Over 60°F.	3	8.8	−5.8
Total	63	63.0	

Source: Greenberg, R. C. 1963. "Two factors influencing the births of mongols to younger mothers." *Med. Off.* 109: 62–64.

of cases during April–October, but it was minimal and could well have been the result of chance alone, particularly since there were only 14 cases, 13 of which were trisomy 21, and one, a translocation. Additional observations in these populations are necessary before any firm conclusions can be drawn. It is of interest that the 2 hospitals had approximately the same incidence of mongolism, even though the mothers in these 2 hospitals differed with respect to socioeconomic status and in the incidence of sex chromatin anomalies.

General Comments

From this review of many studies conducted and reported on in the past 10 years, no clear, consistent pattern of temporo-spatial clustering or of seasonal distribution emerges. Perhaps differences in the methods of study, in the ascertainment of cases, and in the selective reporting of an unusual series of chance circumstances in a particular locality, or the combination of all are responsible for the suggestive presence of clusters. But more extensive population studies in which data are obtained in a systematic, uniform manner from several geographical areas will have to be carried out in order to insure the proper evaluation of these hypotheses, which is not possible at present. The desirability of conducting these studies is indicated by the many observations on the role of viruses in the production of chromosomal abnormalities, a subject recently reviewed by Nichols. Several different types of viruses have been found to produce single chromosomal breaks, pulverization of chromosomes, cell fusions and spindle abnormalities.

4:

Maternal and Prenatal Factors

As a result of the marked association of mongolism with maternal age and the demonstrated relationships between prenatal events and congenital malformations in general, interest has been focused on the role of these factors in the etiology of mongolism. Maternal health, reproductive, hormonal, and constitutional factors, as well as prenatal events, have all been studied.

Menstrual History

Øster (1953) reported an earlier age of menarche and a later age of menopause in a group of mothers of mongols. However, for comparative purposes, he used data collected by other investigators several years before his study of mongols, which of course immediately raises the issue of data comparability. Smith and Record (1955*b*), in a fairly well controlled study, did not confirm these results. More recently, Sigler, Cohen, Lilienfeld, Westlake, and Hetznecker also failed to show any differences between the mothers of mongols and a comparable control group in many of the aspects of menstrual history (Table 4–1).

Reproductive Performance

Several studies have been conducted on the maternal reproductive performance prior to the birth of the mongol child. These are of special interest because it is possible that there is a group of mothers who have a high risk for meiotic nondisjunction. In view of the high frequency of chromosomal abnormalities found among abortions

Table 4–1. Menstrual History of Mothers of Children with Down's Syndrome and of Control Children

Menstrual history	Down's syndrome Number (216)	Controls Number (216)	*P* value
Mean age at menarche (years)	13.56	13.44	.412
Mean age at menopause (years)	45.21	45.93	.276
Still menstruating (per cent)	70.60	77.60	.101
Operative menopause (per cent)	39.30	38.30	.907
Always regular period (per cent)	87.50	87.00	.878
Consulting physician for menstrual difficulty (per cent)	17.10	10.70	.060
Mean duration of menstrual period (days)	5.72	5.54	.204
Mean interval between periods (days)	28.96	28.90	.741

Source: Sigler, A. T., Cohen, B. H., Lilienfeld, A. M., Westlake, J., & Hetznecker, W. H. 1967. "Reproductive and marital experience of parents of children with Down's syndrome (mongolism)." *J. Pediat.* 70: 608–14.

(Chapter 2), this high-risk group should show an increased frequency of monosomic and trisomic conceptions, either by reduced fertility or by increased frequency of fetal loss.

Øster (1953), in his study of 526 mongol families, reported a greater frequency of "abortions" (16.5 per cent) after the birth of the mongol child than before (9.7 per cent). He also demonstrated a longer interval between marriage and the birth of the first child, a mongol, as compared to a first-born who was normal, and a longer pregnancy-free interval before the birth of a mongol as compared with the interval between normal births preceding a mongol birth, taking into account birth order. However, Øster had no control group for comparison and, therefore, it is impossible to evaluate his results.

In 1955, Smith and Record (1955*b*) critically reviewed all of the published literature on this subject and concluded that all of the previous studies had been inadequately controlled. They, in turn, studied a group of 252 mongol children born during 1942–52 in Birmingham, England. Information on mothers' reproductive histories was completed for 217 cases, which was then compared with that for 136 control mothers matched by maternal age. The 136 were all of the mothers who could be traced and interviewed from a matched group of 216 births; this problem created a deficiency in the "40 and over" maternal age group. No differences in fertility experience were noted between marriage and the conception of, or after the conception of, a mongol child. The incidence of abortions was found to be more frequent among mothers of the mongol group when compared with the controls (10.7 per cent as compared to 6.7 per cent). Unfortunately, despite a rather careful statistical analysis of the data, it is difficult to evaluate the results because of the differential ascertainment of the mongol and control mothers as previously noted; this may have introduced a bias in the results.

Ingalls, Babbott, and Philbrook reviewed the obstetric records of mothers of mongol births during the period 1935–54 at one hospital in Boston and compared them with those of a control group, matched for age of the mother of the mongol (Table 4–2). Clearly, there are no differences in fertility between the cases and controls. However, it is of interest that the interval between the birth of a mongol child and a live-born sibling was longer for the cases than for the controls; this results from the fact that 12 of the 31 older mothers of mongol babies had miscarriages prior to the birth of the mongol, as compared to 5 of the 31 age-matched controls. Ingalls, Babbott, and Philbrook also reported that of the total pregnancies prior to the mongol birth, the case mothers had 15.5 per cent terminating in miscarriages or stillbirths and the controls only 9.4 per cent; and 22.1 per cent of multiparous mothers of mongols gave a history of a miscarriage in the first pregnancy, as compared to 10 per cent of the controls.

Lunn, in a survey of 117 mongol children and controls in Glasgow, also obtained information on the reproductive experience of the mothers. He noted that the mothers of the mongols had a total of 509 pregnancies, as compared to 462 in the control group. No difference in frequency of abortions was noted—9.6 per cent as compared to 11.7 per cent.

Table 4–2. Interval between Birth of Mongoloid or Control and Preceding Birth, by 2 Age Groups

	Age group			
	33 years or younger		34 years or older	
	Interval to preceding live birth, stillbirth, or miscarriage (years)	Interval to preceding live birth (years)	Interval to preceding live birth, stillbirth, or miscarriage (years)	Interval to preceding live birth (years)
Mothers of mongols	3.0	4.5	3.6	4.9
Mothers of comparison group	3.0	3.0	4.3	4.5

Source: Ingalls, T. H., Babbott, J., & Philbrook, R. 1957. "The mothers of mongoloid babies: A retrospective appraisal of their health during pregnancy." *Amer. J. Obstet. Gynec.* 74: 572–81.

Coppen and Cowie analyzed the abortion histories of 55 mothers of mongols and reported an unusually high rate of fetal loss among conceptions prior to the birth of the mongol (31 per cent); unfortunately, there was no control group for comparison. Cowie and Slater observed a higher rate of miscarriages after age 35 among mothers who gave birth to a mongol after 37 years of age, as compared to those who gave birth to mongols before the age of 37 years. Again, no comparison group was used except an internal one and, therefore, one hesitates to evaluate these results. Beolchini, Bariatti, and Morganti, in their study of mongol children and controls, also analyzed the reproductive performance of the mothers and found no difference between the case and control groups with respect to (1) average number of conceptions, (2) interval between marriage and birth of mongol or control child, (3) interval between previous pregnancy and birth of mongol or control. However, they did observe a higher frequency of abortions prior to the birth of the mongol child—17.2 per cent as compared to 13.7 per cent among controls. When the mothers were subdivided by maternal age at the time of birth of the index child, the significant differences were observed for those mothers under 40 years of age; no differences were noted for those 40 years of age and over. These results are in direct contrast to those of Cowie and Slater. Stark, in his study of mongol and control children, reported an excess frequency of miscarriages among the mothers of mongols (47 per cent), as compared to control mothers (27 per cent). When maternal age was considered, this difference was essentially found among the mothers who were over 35 years of age at the time of birth of the mongol.

The results of these 3 studies are interesting in light of the suggested relationship with abortion frequency. However, it is necessary in studies of abortion frequencies to take into account the age when the abortions occur, i.e., to determine the maternal age-specific abortion rate. Recently, this has been done in several well-controlled studies. Buck, Valentine, and Hamilton reported on the reproductive performance of mothers of 110 mongol families and 100 control families who were friends of the parents of the mongols and had no retarded children of their own. They analyzed the fertility and fetal-loss rate among these families in considerable detail and compared the pregnancy rates of mothers of mongols and controls within specified age periods because of the relation between age and fertility. The authors also considered the number of years of exposure to conception during specified age periods, and age at marriage was accounted for in the analysis. They calculated the expected number of pregnancies among mothers of mongols, specific for age at marriage and duration of pregnancy exposure in each age period, based on the experience of the control mothers.

Table 4–3 shows their comparison of the observed and expected numbers of pregnancies. The similarity between observed and expected numbers is apparent throughout and in the specific age groups. They noted that among the mothers who had the mongol at 38 years or more, the total fertility considerably exceeds the expected; a result primarily of the greater than expected number of pregnancies in the oldest maternal age group. Apparently, the mongol child of the mother of advanced age is the result of an extra pregnancy rather than of a delayed pregnancy, an observation also made by Ingalls, Babbott, and Philbrook.

Table 4–4 presents the fetal-loss rates as a per cent of the number of pregnancies occurring during 3 specified periods of reproductive life. In the control mothers, 13.2 per cent of pregnancies occurring between the ages of 17 and 27 resulted in fetal loss. For the age groups 28 through 37 and 38 and over, the loss rates were 15.8 per cent and 12.5 per cent, respectively. In this table, fetal-loss rates in each period of life have been subdivided according to the age at which the mongol was born. Buck, Valentine, and Hamilton point out that, "The comparison of the rates of fetal loss in mothers of mongols and control women offers no evidence that the former have, throughout their reproductive period, an abnormal risk of non-disjunction." How-

Table 4–3. Observed and Expected Numbers of Pregnancies for Mothers of Mongols in Specific Maternal Age Periods by Age at Birth of Mongol

	Age at birth of mongol					
	17–27		28–37		38+	
Age period	Observed	Expected	Observed	Expected	Observed	Expected
17–27	70	61	59	69	19	26
28–37	24	31	114	98	69	55
38+	2	2	16	15	61	20
Total	96	94	189	182	149	101

Source: Buck, C., Valentine, G. H., & Hamilton, K. 1966. "Reproductive performance of mothers of mongols." *Amer. J. Ment. Defic.* 70: 886–94.

Table 4–4. Fetal Losses per 100 Pregnancies in Mothers of Mongols and in Control Mothers

Maternal age period		Mothers of mongols by age at birth of mongol			Control mothers
		17–27	28–37	38+	
17–27	Pregnancies	40	59	19	190
	Losses	8	7	0	25
	Per cent loss	20.0	11.9	0.0	13.2
28–37	Pregnancies	24	66	69	139
	Losses	4	13	11	22
	Per cent loss	16.7	19.7	15.9	15.8
38+	Pregnancies	2	16	29	8
	Losses	0	2	8	1
	Per cent loss	0.0	12.5	27.6	12.5

Note: Pregnancies exclude the mongol birth.

Source: Buck, C., Valentine, G. H., & Hamilton, K. 1966. "Reproductive performance of mothers of mongols." *Amer. J. Ment. Defic.* 70: 886–94.

ever, upon closer examination of this table an interesting observation does emerge. The fetal loss rates are highest in the maternal age periods during which the mongols were born; the rates are highest along the diagonals of the table. A suggestive explanation for this observation is that the mother may be exposed to an etiological agent for both mongolism and fetal loss during the same time period.

There is apparently an excessive rate of fetal loss at ages 38 and over among mothers whose mongol was born while in that age group. However, the small numbers in the control group and the discrepancy between their fetal-loss rate and that found by Shapiro, Jones, and Densen support the possibility that this difference may be an overestimate.

Sigler, Cohen, Lilienfeld, Westlake, and Hetznecker, in their study of 216 mongols and controls, also analyzed the reproductive history of the mothers. No significant differences were found in the number of pregnancies, abortions or stillbirths either before or after the birth of the index mongol or control child (Table 4–5). No important differences were noted in the interval of time between the preceding pregnancy and the birth of the index child, or in the interval of time following the index child's birth and subsequent pregnancies. In addition, the number of neonatal and childhood deaths in the siblings of the mongol children and controls was very similar: 95.6 per cent of the siblings with mongolism and 95.2 per cent of the controls were alive at the time of the study.

Matsunaga (1967*b*) reported on the pregnancy-free interval prior to the birth of 223 mongol children, as compared to a group of con-

Table 4–5. Pregnancy Wastage in Mothers of Children with Down's Syndrome and in Mothers of Controls by Maternal Age and by Time Relationship to Index Child

Maternal age groups	Prior to index child				Subsequent to index child			
	Total pregnancies		Abortions and stillbirths (per cent)		Total pregnancies		Abortions and stillbirths (per cent)	
	Down's	Controls	Down's	Controls	Down's	Controls	Down's	Controls
15–19	1	4	100.0	0	10	16	10.0	0
20–24	32	36	25.0	19.9	52	64	11.5	18.8
25–29	43	57	16.3	17.6	41	47	9.7	23.4
30–34	127	105	15.8	14.3	44	32	20.5	9.4
35–39	185	167	15.7	14.4	28	24	28.6	12.5
40–44	135	148	13.3	13.6	1	5	0	40.0
45–49	4	0	25.0	0	0	0	0	0
50+	0	0	0	0	0	0	0	0
Total	527	517	15.9	14.7	176	188	15.9	16.5

Note: For prior to index child, P value $> .30$ for stillbirths and abortions. Subsequent to index child, P value $> .80$ for stillbirths and abortions.

Source: Sigler, A. T., Cohen, B. H., Lilienfeld, A. M., Westlake, J., & Hetznecker, W. H. 1967. "Reproductive and marital experience of parents of children with Down's syndrome (mongolism)." *J. Pediat.* 70: 608–14.

trols matched for sex, year of birth, maternal age, and live-birth order (Table 4–6). No differences are noted even after a more sensitive analysis of paired differences: the mean difference of pairs of cases and controls was 0.005 years with a standard deviation of 0.097.

It would appear that in those studies which have been adequately controlled, no differences in fertility and fetal loss are found between the mothers of mongol children and control mothers. Admittedly, in each of these studies the number of cases may be inadequate to detect small differences and, therefore, if differences do exist they probably are modest. Since all of these studies are of surviving mongols, and if, as Buck, Valentine, and Hamilton suggested, there is a relationship between early death of a mongol and prior reproductive performance of the mother of a mongol, there is a real need for a more intensive investigation of this issue; one requiring a study of newborn mongols.

Exposure to Ionizing Radiation

In view of the well-established relationship between ionizing radiation and chromosomal abnormalities in humans, the relationship of ionizing radiation and leukemia, and the experimental production of nondisjunction by radiation, investigators became especially interested in determining whether parents of mongols had had an excessive ex-

Table 4–6. Distribution of the Interval Free from Pregnancy before the Births of Infants with Down's Syndrome and Controls Matched by Sex, Year of Birth, Maternal Age, and Live-Birth Rank

Pregnancy-free interval (months)	Cases		Controls	
	Number	Per cent	Number	Per cent
Very brief (0–12)	30	13.5	33	14.8
Brief (13–24)	90	40.4	82	36.8
Intermediate (25–48)	75	33.6	84	37.7
Long (49 and over)	28	12.6	24	10.8
Total	223	100.1	223	100.1
Mean interval (months)	31.0		31.0	

Source: Matsunaga, E. 1967*b*. "Parental age, live-birth order, and pregnancy-free interval in Down's syndrome in Japan," in: Ciba Foundation Study Group No. 25, *Mongolism*, pp. 6–22 (Boston: Little, Brown and Company).

posure to radiation (Schmickel; Cantolino, Schmickel, *et al.*; Mavor; Lilienfeld). Lunn in 1959 reported that the per cent of "significant" histories of X-ray exposure of mothers of 117 mongols did not differ from that of mothers of controls. In 1961, Uchida and Curtis reported that 28 per cent of the mothers of 49 mongols were exposed to 4 or more abdominal X-rays or fluoroscopings as compared to 4 per cent of the mothers of 66 cleft-lip children and 14 per cent of mothers of 44 neighbors. Carter, Evans, and Stewart did not confirm Uchida's results in their study of 51 mongols and 51 matched controls with other congenital malformations. Schull and Neel presented some data from Hiroshima and Nagasaki which failed to indicate any excess in the frequency of mongolism among those exposed to the atomic bombs. Except for the Japanese experience, each of these studies was either primarily concerned with diagnostic radiation experience or did not distinguish between diagnostic and other types of radiation. In addition, each study has limitations of a methodological nature imposed either by the method of control selection, or, as in the study with negative findings, by the number of cases selected, which was not sufficient to adequately test the hypothesis of a small to moderate effect of radiation. The latter objection can also be raised with respect to the Hiroshima–Nagasaki experience.

With these objections in mind, Sigler, Lilienfeld, Cohen, and Westlake (1965*a*) conducted a well-controlled study in Baltimore, where they compared the parents of 216 mongol children with the parents of a "control group" of normal children carefully matched for hospital of birth (or birth at home), date of birth, sex, and maternal age at birth. The parents of both groups were interviewed (those who refused, about an equal number in each group, were excluded from the study) and the questions were phrased to omit any reference to the child. The parents' names were submitted to all Baltimore hospitals in an effort to locate existing medical records which (if found) were thoroughly scrutinized.

There were no significant differences between the groups in their residential history, the number of hospital admissions, or the place where they had received the radiation. Most of the exposures had taken place in private clinics or doctors' offices, rather than in hospitals, and the hospital records were primarily used as a check on the comparability of the groups.

Radiation exposures were divided into diagnostic (excluding fluoroscopy), fluoroscopic, therapeutic, and occupational; the 2 groups did not differ significantly except for fluoroscopic and therapeutic exposures (Table 4–7). Among the mothers of mongol children, 17.7 per cent had had one or more fluoroscopic exposures before the child was born, but only 8.1 per cent of the control mothers; 14.5 per cent of the mothers of mongol children had been exposed to radiotherapy

Table 4–7. Summary of Parental Diagnostic, Fluoroscopic and Therapeutic Radiation (One or More Exposures), Interview, and Medical Records Prior to Birth of the Index Child

	Mothers				Fathers			
	Mongols		Controls		Mongols		Controls	
Type of exposure	Number	Per cent	Number	Per cent	Number	Per cent	Number	Per cent
No Radiation	104	50.0	124	59.9	86	43.7	102	50.0
Radiation								
Diagnostic only	50	24.0	56	27.1	62	31.5	52	25.5
Fluoroscopic only	10	4.8	7	3.4	11	5.6	11	5.4
Therapeutic only	8	3.3	3	1.4	4	2.0	4	1.9
Diagnostic and fluoroscopic	14	6.7	8	3.9	17	8.6	21	10.3
Diagnostic and therapeutic	7	3.4	6	2.9	11	5.6	10	4.9
Fluoroscopic and therapeutic	2	1.0	1	0.5	2	1.0	2	1.0
Diagnostic, fluoroscopic and therapeutic	13	6.3	2	0.9	4	2.0	2	1.0
Total known	208		207		197		204	
Unknown	8	3.7	9	4.2	19	8.8	12	5.6
Total	216		216		216		216	

Source: Sigler, A. T., Lilienfeld, A. M., Cohen, B. H., & Westlake, J. E. 1965*a*. "Radiation exposure in parents of children with mongolism (Down's syndrome)." *Bull. Johns Hopkins Hosp.* 117: 374–99.

(8.8 per cent for skin conditions), compared with 5.1 per cent of the control mothers (2.3 per cent for skin conditions). The skin conditions treated in many of the first group were acne and eczema, but none of the control mothers were treated for these—an unexplained finding.

Though no difference was found between the groups in occupational exposure to ionizing radiation, 2 interesting differences did emerge: (1) 7.9 per cent of the mothers of mongols had been employed in the medical field, compared with 3.3 per cent of the controls, and exposure was possible; and (2) a slight difference in the military history of the fathers in the 2 groups led to the finding that 8.7 per cent of the fathers of the mongols had worked with radar, as compared to 3.2 per cent in the control group; this was the only significant difference between the 2 groups of fathers. This study showed that for all kinds of ionizing radiation, 50 per cent of the mothers in the mongol group had never been exposed at all, compared with 60 per cent of those in the control group; while 13 mothers in the mongol group, but only 2 in the control group, had been exposed to more than one kind (diagnostic, fluoroscopic, therapeutic) of radiation. All these differences are significant, at the 5 per cent level at least.

The results reported by Sigler, Lilienfeld, Cohen, and Westlake (1965*a*), as well as the experimental data, are suggestive of a relationship between radiation and mongolism. Confirmation of these results, however, for both ionizing radiation and radar exposure is necessary.

Maternal Ill Health during Pregnancy

For reasons already mentioned, several investigators have studied the possible relationship of mongolism to different states of maternal ill health during pregnancy. This was reviewed by Ingalls in a series of reports published during 1947–57 (Ingalls, Babbott, & Philbrook; Ingalls & Gordon; Ingalls, 1947*b*). A seemingly high frequency of bleeding during pregnancy has been reported by several authors (Biedleman; Benda, 1946; Ingalls, Babbott, & Philbrook). Typical of the results was that of Ingalls, Babbott, and Philbrook, who reported a 20 per cent frequency of bleeding during the first trimester as compared to 10 per cent in a control group. Many of these studies were inadequately controlled, particularly with regard to maternal age. Smith and Record (1955*b*), in a better controlled study, found no statistically significant difference in the frequency of uterine bleeding.

Some investigators have also suggested that gynecological disorders are more frequent among mothers of mongols than among those of controls (Ingalls, Babbott, & Philbrook). Smith and Record (1955*b*) found no such relationship in their study. Ingalls, Babbott, and Philbrook also reported a higher frequency of organic heart disease among the mothers of mongols than among controls (30 per cent versus 10 per cent).

Related to these studies are the reports by Stott and Drillien and Wilkinson indicating a higher frequency of history of emotional shock among mothers during the mongol pregnancies as compared to pregnancies of non-mongol mental defectives. These studies are open to criticism, since the information was obtained retrospectively and no doubt there is a considerable degree of error in this type of data. However, in view of the possible existence of a relationship between the nervous and endocrine systems and the possible influence of the latter on mongolism, the potential role of emotional factors should not be dismissed. A thorough investigation of this factor requires a prospective study.

Many of these findings should now be reinterpreted in the light of the cytogenetic findings which indicate essentially that any influence on nondisjunction should occur prior to, or at about, the time of conception, or at the very latest, shortly after conception. In addition, since most of these studies have not been adequately controlled for maternal age, it is quite possible that many of the findings merely reflect the increased frequency of these conditions with maternal age, or some may even be a result, rather than a cause, of the mongol pregnancy.

Maternal Exposure to Fluorides in the Water Supply

Based on the clinical observations of a paucity of dental caries among mongol children, Rapaport hypothesized that an increased fluoride concentration in the water supply was of etiological importance in mongolism (Benda, 1960; Rapaport). To test this hypothesis, he collected data on the frequency of mongol births in cities in Illinois, selected on the basis of the fluoride concentration of the water supply. Using birth and death certificates and "registries of specialized medical schools in the state," he ascertained all of the cases of mongolism born from January 1, 1950 to December 31, 1956 for mothers who had resided before the birth of the mongol in cities of from 10,000 to 100,000 population in Illinois. He then determined the frequency of mongolism for groups of cities, according to the fluoride concentration of their water supply. The results are presented in Table 4–8.

The data in this table are interpreted by Rapaport as suggesting an increase in the incidence rate of mongolism with increasing fluoride concentration. Unfortunately, the data are difficult to evaluate since the total frequency of mongolism is 0.44 per 1,000 births, a much lower rate than those presented in Chapter 2. This low rate suggests a relatively high degree of incomplete ascertainment of cases, which in turn raises additional questions. There is the possible influence of bias in the ascertainment of cases and, of course, there may well have been a differential and biased ascertainment in cities with different fluoride concentrations in their water supply. Although fluorides in the water supply may be of etiological significance, the results of Rapaport's analysis are inadequate to substantiate that hypothesis.

Other Maternal Factors

Cowie (1961), in a small series of mothers, reported that mothers of mongols who were under 27 years of age had higher androgyny scores and higher biacromial diameters than mothers over 27 years of age. They also found that these young mothers had an increased output of urinary dehydroepiandrostrone; more than that of both a control group and older mothers (Rundle, Coppen, & Cowie). This confirmed previous findings of Ek and Jensen and suggests that endocrinological abnormalities may be characteristic of mothers of mongols. Clearly this should be studied in a larger series of cases.

Table 4–8. Frequency of Mongolism in Cities of 10,000–100,000 Population, Illinois, January 1, 1950–December 31, 1956

Concentration of fluoride in water supply (mg./lit.)	Number of cities	Number of births	Cases of mongolism	
			Number	Incidence rate (per 100,000 births)
0.0	15	63,521	15	23.61
0.1–0.2	24	132,665	52	39.20
0.3–0.7	17	70,111	33	47.07
1.0–2.6	12	67,053	48	71.59

Note: Statistical significance: $X^2 = 16.29$, $P < .001$.

Source: Rapaport, I. 1963. "Mongolian oligophrenia and dental caries." *Rev. Stomat.* 64: 207–18.

For many years there has been suggestive and conflicting evidence on the frequency of thyroid abnormalities among mothers of mongols. Clinico-epidemiological studies of this relationship were reviewed by Ek; unfortunately, most of the studies were inadequately controlled. Ek studied 41 mothers of mongols during 1956–57; these women were examined and had blood samples collected for protein blood iodine (PBI) determinations. He reported a mean value for this group of women that was significantly higher than the normal values in his laboratory. In addition, he reported a high frequency of goiter in these women (29 per cent), which was higher than the normal expectancy (1.1 per cent). Unfortunately, here too there was no control group.

Reflecting this interest in the relationship of thyroid disease to mongolism and the more recent emerging interest in autoimmunity in the etiology of disease, Fialkow (1967) reported that 29 per cent of 242 mothers of mongol patients showed evidence of thyroid antibodies, as compared to 16 per cent of a group of controls who were age and sex matched. Additional analysis indicated that the difference is essentially limited to mothers under 35 years of age (Table 4–9). This suggests that this relationship might be more significant in the more unusual type of chromosomal abnormalities in mongolism—mosaic, translocation, and familial trisomy 21 and has been supported by some incomplete data on 4 mosaic mongols, 3 of whom had mothers with evidence of thyroid disease.

Table 4–9. Observed and Expected Positive Thyroid Antibody Tests in Mothers of Children with Down's Syndrome in Relation to Maternal Age at Birth of the Propositus

Maternal age						
At test (years)	18–32	33–45	46–70	All ages		
Expectation of positive test	0.030	0.144	0.291	0.161	Number of positive reactions	
At birth	Number of mothers tested (number positive)				Expected	Observed
15–19	5 (1)	2 (1)	0 (0)	7	0.438	2
20–24	23 (4)	1 (0)	1 (0)	25	1.125	4
25–29	25 (9)	18 (4)	1 (0)	44	3.633	13
30–34	13 (4)	21 (8)	10 (3)	44	6.324	15
35–39		31 (7)	24 (5)	55	11.448	12
40–44		22 (7)	29 (11)	51	11.607	18
45–49		2 (0)	14 (5)	16	4.362	5
Total	66	97	79	242	38.937	69

Source: Fialkow, P. J. 1967. "Thyroid antibodies, Down's syndrome, and maternal age." *Nature* 214: 1253–54.

However, similar observations were made by Dallaire and Flynn (1967*b*) in a study of 44 mothers of trisomy 21 children and several comparison groups, including 51 mothers of children with multiple malformations but normal chromosomal patterns, 50 mothers of normal children; a group of 120 women between 19 and 69 years of age who had no children; and 6 mothers of children with chromosomal abnormalities other than trisomy 21 (Table 4–10). From these data, it is quite clear that there is a significant increase in the per cent of positive sera (for thyroglobulin) among mothers of mongols, as compared to the other groups of mothers.

Interpretation of these data is not clear at present. The following hypotheses can be entertained to explain these observations: (1) an increase in antibodies produces an increase in the risk of chromosomal abnormalities resulting in mongolism; (2) the mongol fetus stimulates the mother to develop antibodies; and (3) both mongolism and increased antibodies may be a result of a common factor. Evaluation of these hypotheses would require a prospective study, which will be discussed later in recommending further epidemiologic research.

In addition, Allison and Paton have suggested that maternal infection with *Mycoplasma hominis* type 1 may be of etiologic importance in mongolism (Allison). They point out that the frequency of antibodies to this mycoplasma increases with increasing age, mycoplasma infects the entire genital tract from the ovary to the vagina and produces hydrogen peroxide which can cause chromosomal abnormalities. In tissue culture the *Mycoplasma hominis* type 1 produces endoduplica-

Table 4–10. Frequency of Positive Test for Thyroid Antibody and Other Characteristics of Mothers of Aneuploid Children and Controls

Group	Number of women tested	Mean number: Pregnancies	Mean number: Miscarriages	Mean number: Normal siblings	Mean birth order	Positive tanned red cell: Number	Positive tanned red cell: Per cent	Mean age (at proband's birth)	Mean age (at test)
Down's syndrome	44	3.77	0.54	2.13	3.45	12	27.3	33.25	34.90
All aneuploid	50	3.86	0.50	2.28	3.56	13	26.0	33.08	34.70
Multiple malformations	51	4.05	0.45	2.78	3.60	6	11.7	28.47	31.80
Normal controls	50	3.10	0	2.10	3.10	6	12.0	20.60	34.24
Gravida-O women	120	0	0	0	0	3	2.5	—	41.32

Source: Dallaire, L. & Flynn, D. 1967*b*. "Frequency of antibodies to thyroglobulin in relation to gravidity and to Down's syndrome." *Canad. Med. Assoc. J.* 97: 209–12.

tions and chromosomal abnormalities. Studies are now in progress comparing the antibody status of mothers of mongols and controls and their results will be of interest.

Of some interest is the finding of Sigler, Cohen, Lilienfeld, Westlake, and Hetznecker of a significantly greater number of multiple marriages before the birth of a mongol child than that in a normal control group (16.2 per cent of multiple marriages as compared to 6.9 per cent). Other aspects of marital history did not differ in the 2 groups (Table 4–11). These results are puzzling and require confirmation.

Table 4–11. Marital and Reproductive History of Mothers of Children with Down's Syndrome and of Control Children

Marital and reproductive history	Down's syndrome Number (216)	Controls Number (216)	*P* value
Married twice or more before birth of index child (per cent)	16.2	6.9	<.01
Married once or more following birth of index child (per cent)	1.4	0.5	>.30
Median number of years married before birth of index child	8.13	8.48	>.30
Median number of years married before first pregnancy ended	1.93	1.99	>.50
Median interval between previous pregnancy and birth of index child	2.93	3.21	>.50

Source: Sigler, A. T., Cohen, B. H., Lilienfeld, A. M., Westlake, J., & Hetznecker, W. H. 1967. "Reproductive and marital experience of parents of children with Down's syndrome (mongolism)." *J. Pediat*. 70: 608–14.

5:

Familial Aggregation and Twin Studies

Familial Aggregation of Mongolism

Before chromosomal abnormalities were implicated in mongolism, familial occurrence was a major area of research interest. Two aspects of familial aggregation held particular interest for the investigators—the frequency of mongolism among sibs of mongols and the risk of the birth of a second mongol; the latter attracted attention because of the practicality of genetic counseling. Böök and Reed, recalculating data presented earlier by Penrose (1934–35), found that among the 814 siblings of 217 persons with mongolism, 7, or 0.85 per cent, were mongoloid. Later, Penrose (1939) reported a frequency of 1.47 per cent among 271 siblings of mongols; these risks did not appear to be excessive. Additional computations of the Penrose data show that among 153 children born alive subsequent to the first mongol child, 6, or 3.9 per cent, were also mongoloid.

By 1956, Øster had collected from the literature approximately 30 well-documented cases of multiple occurrence of mongolism in siblings. In an analysis of his own data, he reported that the mothers of 526 mongols had 343 additional live births, 4 of whom were mongols; a contrast to the expected number of 1.4, which was not statistically significant.

In 1961, Carter and Evans reviewed some of the methodological problems that had not been considered in earlier studies but which may well have been responsible for some bias in the estimates. They collected family data on 642 patients of a hospital in London, during the period 1944–55, and combined these data with those of Øster (1956). They analyzed the frequency of mongolism among sibs who were younger and older than the index mongol child by maternal age, and it became clear that there was a significant increase in the risk of having a second mongol child (Table 5–1). There were 9 affected younger sibs as compared to an expectancy of less than 3. One also notes from this table that among younger mothers, the observed/expected ratio is quite high, with a gradual decrease in ratio as the maternal age increases. In judging the risks in terms of the mother's age at the time of birth of the index child, one recognizes that a higher risk prevails among younger mothers (Table 5–2). In the same year, 1961, Berg and Kirman reported similar results from a survey of families of 778 mongols with 367 children born after the birth of the mongol child, who was either living at home or institutionalized in London. A summary of their results is presented in Table 5–3. Note the markedly excessive risk of a second mongol among the younger mothers.

Lejeune, Gautier, and Turpin's (1959*a*) report of trisomy in mongols in 1959 stimulated a great deal of interest in the chromosomal patterns in familial mongolism. Penrose, Ellis, and Delhanty reported on a cytological study of several members of a family with 2 mongol sibs where the patients' mother, maternal grandmother, and sister had 45 chromosomes; this was interpreted as a reciprocal translocation, an interpretation suggested by Snell and Picken's experimental work on hereditary malformations in mice. Carter, Hamerton, Polani, Gunalp, and Weller and Polani, Ford, Briggs, and Clarke reported similar types of families. Finally, Hamerton, Briggs, Giannelli, and Carter performed chromosomal studies on the families of 9 index patients

Table 5–1. Relative Prevalence of Down's Syndrome in Sibs of Index Patients and in General Population

	Maternal age at birth of sib				
	15–24	25–29	30–34	35+	Total
Younger sibs affected	2	4	2	1	9
Expected number affected	0.039	0.112	0.176	1.988	2.315
Observed/expected	51.3	35.7	11.4	0.5	3.9
Older sibs affected	2	2	1	2	7
Expected number affected	0.370	0.578	0.730	1.850	3.527
Observed/expected	5.4	3.5	1.4	1.1	2.0

Note: Carter and Evans' series and Øster's series combined.

Source: Carter, C. O. & Evans, K. A. 1961. "Risk of parents who have had one child with Down's syndrome (mongolism) having another child similarly affected." *Lancet* 2: 785–88.

Table 5–2. Comparison of Observed and Expected Number of Affected Sibs According to Mother's Age at Birth of Index Patient

	Maternal age group			
	15–24	25–34	35+	Total
Observed affected sibs	4	3	2	9
Expected affected sibs				
A	0.068	0.606	1.741	2.415
B	0.108	0.602	1.646	2.356
Observed/expected				
A	58.8	5.0	1.1	3.7
B	37.0	5.0	1.2	3.8

Note: A, estimated from the incidence of mongolism reported by Carter & MacCarthy (1951). *B*, estimated by comparing the maternal age distribution for the cases with that for England and Wales.

Source: Carter, C. O. & Evans, K. A. 1961. "Risk of parents who have had one child with Down's syndrome (mongolism) having another child similarly affected." *Lancet* 2: 785–88.

with an affected sib using the series of cases reported on earlier by Carter and Evans. In 3 of these families translocations were found, and in all of these families the mother was under 25 years of age at the birth of the index patient. Investigators seem to agree that the chromosomal composition of these families accounted for most of the increased risk for young mothers of a mongol child to have a second affected child.

Gradually one saw the development of the concept that familial translocation represented the principal source of multiple cases of mongolism in a family. Many investigators began to study the chromosomes of families where there was a familial occurrence of mongolism, and in light of the previously determined maternal age relationships, many of the studies were limited to families of young mothers (Atkins, O'Sullivan, *et al.*; Dekaban, Bender, & Economos; Breg, Miller, & Schmickel; Shaw; Forssman & Lehmann). A detailed consideration of these problems would require detailed cytological

Table 5–3. Increased Risk of Having a Second Child with Mongolism

Maternal age at birth of subsequent child (years)	Number of live births after birth of mongol	Expected incidence of mongolism in subsequent births if risk is not increased	Incidence of mongolism in subsequent births	Risk increased by
<40	286	0.56	4	7.1×
40+	81	1.34	3	2.2×
Total	367	1.90	7	3.7×

Source: Berg, J. M. & Kirman, B. H. 1961. "Risk of dual occurrence of mongolism in sibships." *Arch. Dis. Child.* 36: 645–48.

descriptions and there are several excellent recently published reviews in this area; therefore, it did not seem appropriate to present the detailed genetic and cytological data in a discussion of the epidemiology of mongolism (Penrose & Smith; Hamerton). However, to provide an over-all idea of the relative magnitude of these types of mongols, we have reproduced a table from a paper by Day and Wright summarizing the types of data obtained in a series of such studies (Table 5–4). We note that in these young mothers, only 11 per cent of the mongols are due to translocations and of the 12 cases reported, 3, or 25 per cent, can be said to be inherited, that is, a parent has been identified as a translocation carrier; the inherited group represents about 3 per cent of all the mongols in these series. In summarizing these data, the authors indicate that

> the value of chromosomal studies in Down's syndrome can be illustrated in the following way. By combining the 41 patients reported here with those discussed in similar studies (Table 5–4), 3 of the 109 patients (1 in 36) are shown to have received their extra number 21 material from a parent known to carry a translocation. In all 3 patients the translocation was of the D/G type, and the mother was the carrier. The risk of recurrence in subsequent offspring of a D/G translocation carrier mother

Table 5–4. Distribution of Chromosomal Abnormalities in Several Series of Patients with Down's Syndrome by Maternal Ages at Parturition and by Type and Frequency of Translocation

Investigator and year of report	Maternal age	Chromosomal abnormality: Trisomy 21	Translocation D/G	Translocation G/G	Total	Inherited translocations	Total patients	Translocation frequency: All	Translocation frequency: Inherited
Hayashi (1963)	<30	28	3	0	3	1	31	0.10	0.33
Breg, Miller, & Schmickel (1962)	<29	10	2	0	2	1	12	0.17	0.50
Edwards, Dent, & Guli (1963)	<30	21	2	2	4	0	25	0.16	0.00
Subtotal		59	7	2	9	2	68	0.13	0.22
Day & Wright (1965)	<20	38	1	2	3	1	41	0.07	0.33
Total		97	8	4	12	3	109	0.11	0.25

Note: Trisomy 21 includes mosaics, 46/47, 2–21/3–21. Inherited translocation frequency refers to those inherited from an identified carrier parent.

Source: Day, R. W. & Wright, S. W. 1965. "Down's syndrome at young maternal ages: Chromosomal and family studies." *J. Pediat.* 66: 764–71.

can be estimated at 1 in 3. If chromosomal studies are not performed, the recurrence risk can be estimated by combining the 2 fractions, $\frac{1}{36}$ (for the proportion of patients with an inherited translocation) times $\frac{1}{3}$ (the recurrence risk to a D/G translocation carrier mother). The result, $\frac{1}{108}$, or approximately 1 per cent, gives an estimate of the empiric risk or chance that a mother less than 30 years old at the birth of her first affected infant might have another child with Down's syndrome in any succeeding pregnancy.

When chromosomal studies have been performed, however, a patient is identified as having either trisomy or a translocation. The recurrence risk in the former is small, certainly much less than 1 per cent. If a translocation is found, the recurrence risk is higher. However, a large proportion (three-fourths in these data) of translocations arise *de novo.* Demonstration of normal parental complements will provide evidence on this point. Finally, if the patient has a D/G translocation shown to be inherited from a carrier mother, the recurrence risk is probably high, estimated here at 1 in 3.

The above calculations are based on a small sample of patients. It must be reaffirmed that all these figures are open to modification, i.e., the risk changed according to the type of translocation and the sex of the carrier parent. For instance, a sample which included inherited G/G translocations or identified parental carriers might yield very different risk figures (Lejeune). Further, none of the estimates given should apply to families with a history of Down's syndrome; here chromosomal studies are strongly indicated. On the other hand, the relative magnitude of differences in these estimated recurrence risks, according to the type of chromosomal abnormality, suggests that such studies in families where the maternal age at birth of the first affected child is less than 30 years have considerable value.

An interesting computation was carried out by Petersen and Luzzatti using these familial data. Given that, (1) 1.8 per cent of mongols born to mothers 15 to 29 years of age is due to the presence of a D/21 translocation in the mothers, and (2) the expected proportion of affected offspring born to such mothers is 0.33, and (3) the overall frequency of mongols in this maternal age group is about 0.7 per 1,000 births, they went on to estimate that in this age group, three-quarters of the increased recurrence risk can be accounted for by a D/21 translocation. In the 30 to 34 maternal age group, this estimate becomes one-half, and for those over 35 there is no increase in recurrence risk due to D/21 translocations. The authors admit that there are certain statistical problems that have not been taken into account in making these estimates, such as the small series of cases on which some of the frequencies are based, the problems associated with the pooling of data, as well as those of ascertainment of cases. However, it is an interesting approach since it does provide some idea of the order of magnitude of the relative importance of certain cytological types.

It is also clear that for the mongol population as a whole, considering the relatively smaller per cent of mongols born to mothers in the younger ages, the contribution of this genetically determined type of mongol, though small, is of great biological and genetic interest.

Familial aggregation of trisomy 21 has also been reported in all maternal age groups. Zellweger indicated that 30 such sibships have been reported and no doubt more exist but have probably escaped recognition since familial studies have been concentrating on the translocation mongols. Investigators have speculated on possible reasons for familial aggregation which suggest familial aggregation of nondisjunction. There is experimental evidence in drosophilia simulans that a rare recessive trait causes nondisjunction at oogenesis (Sturtevant). Some investigators have therefore considered the possibility that a recessive gene influences nondisjunction. If such a gene is sufficiently rare in the population, one should then find a high frequency of consanguineous marriages among parents and/or grandparents of mongols. Forssman and Akesson (1967) in Sweden found that 9, or 0.8 per cent, of the parents of 1,079 cases were related, not a very different frequency from that found in the Swedish population. Analysis of paternal and maternal grandparents indicated that 1.7 per cent of the former and 1.5 per cent of the latter were consanguineous marriages—a frequency which was close to expectancy. The finding of a higher frequency of consanguineous marriages among grandparents than among the parents probably reflects the steadily decreasing frequency of consanguineous marriages in Sweden. The authors also reported on some data they obtained from Penrose in England indicating that less than 1 per cent (5 out of 700) of the parents were consanguineous, as well as the grandparents, a similar order of magnitude. Matsunaga (1966), in a series of 104 Japanese mongols, Berg, in a series of 302 mongols in London, and Polani, in a series of 208 mongols, similarly did not find a higher frequency of consanguineous marriages among parents of mongols. Additional evidence on the influence of consanguinity is available from a study of the prevalence of mongolism in an inbred population. Kwiterovich, Cross, and McKusick reported a prevalence (0.16 per cent) of mongolism in an inbred Old Order Amish community that is essentially the same as that observed in outbred populations. These data suggest that recessive genes are not involved in producing or predisposing to nondisjunctional events leading to mongolism.

It has also been inferred that familial aggregation reflects the presence of undetected gonadal mosaicism of both normal and trisomy 21 cells in these parents. This hypothesis would be difficult to test, although some efforts should be made to do so.

Viewing the matter from another perspective, some investigators are inclined to think that familial aggregation of trisomy is a relatively rare occurrence (Ingalls & Henry). Evaluating this degree of rarity is difficult because of the possible influence the birth of a mongol child may have on the parents' decision to have additional children, an area for which very little information is available.

Other Chromosomal Abnormalities in Families of Mongols

It is of interest from both epidemiological and genetic viewpoints that over a period of many years investigators have reported series of families where mongolism has occurred together with other chromosomal abnormalities. The types of chromosomal abnormalities among sibs, offspring, first cousins, aunts, and nieces have included Turner's syndrome, Klinefelter's syndrome, trisomy 17–18, XXXXY males, XXX females, and others. About 20 such families have been reported and summarized by Penrose and Smith and Hecht, Bryant, Motulsky, and Giblett.

There has been considerable speculation that the familial aggregation of different forms of chromosomal aberrations is of etiological significance and indicates the influence of genetic factors on nondisjunction or of the influence of viral or other agents which aggregate in families. One of the considerations in accepting such an interpretation rests on whether or not the observed degree of familial aggregation is a chance phenomenon. Several investigators have made efforts to clarify this question. For example, Hecht, Bryant, Motulsky, and Giblett surveyed 60 families with trisomy 13–15 or trisomy 18 and found 3 mongol sibs. They estimated from the maternal age incidence data of Carter and MacCarthy that 0.15 sibs would be expected, a difference from the observed number that was highly statistically significant ($P < 0.001$).

However, one of the major difficulties in interpreting such data, including those reported by Hecht, Bryant, Motulsky, and Giblett, is that the problems of ascertainment were not resolved. Apparently, because of the rarity of the condition, many of the families included in these studies were collected from many cities throughout the U.S. and Europe. It is quite possible that families with more than one child affected with these different types of chromosomal abnormalities have a higher probability of being brought to the investigators' attention. Such biased ascertainment would no doubt produce a higher degree of familial aggregation than is actually present, and these data should therefore be cautiously interpreted.

Offspring of Females with Mongolism

Benda, in 1946, stated that "as far as is known, no mongoloid girl had ever become pregnant." Since then there have been reports on 13 cases of mongol females with offspring. These have been summarized by Johnston and Jaslow, and Tricomi, Valenti, and Hall. According to genetic theory, 50 per cent of these children should be mongols and the actual observations are in accord with theoretical expectations.

Twin Studies

Prior to the cytological era, investigators were interested in twin studies in attempting to distinguish between genetic and environmental factors in the etiology of mongolism. The method most frequently used in such studies was to select a group of mongols who are members of a twin pair, determine which twins are monozygotic or dizygotic, and for each of these types, determine the per cent concordance, i.e., the per cent of twins, both members of whom have the disease. If the disease is completely genetically determined, the per cent concordance among monozygotic twins would be 100 per cent, whereas the concordance for dizygotic twins would be of a much lower order of magnitude. On the other hand, a completely environmentally determined disease would result in concordance frequencies that are approximately the same for both types of twins. If a strong genetic component interacts with the environment to produce the disease, the frequency among monozygotes should be less than 100 per cent, but significantly higher than among dizygotes.

The early literature on twin studies of mongolism consists of individual case reports of concordant and discordant twin pairs. Several interested investigators summarized all of the reported cases in the literature and added several of their own cases with an analysis in terms of concordance percentages. This procedure posed several methodological problems. Many of the early individual case reports diagnosed zygosity on a clinical basis, the validity of which is open to question. This method could, of course, bias the results if the presence of the same disease in both members of a twin pair influenced the investigator in making a monozygotic diagnosis. Another consideration is the possibility that individual case reports are not a representative sample of all cases of mongol twins in the population. The more unusual cases, such as a monozygotic twin or concordant twins, probably have a greater chance of being reported. The possibility of such selective factors limits the inferences that may be derived from such data.

The most recently reported summary of case reports in the literature is that of DeWolff, Schärer, and Lejeune in 1962 (Table 5–5). This summary includes one monozygotic twin pair on whom a chromosomal analysis was done; one member of the pair was a standard mongol whereas the other was chromosomally and phenotypically normal. This could occur from an abnormal division of the chromosomes during the early stages of development.

Allen and Baroff reported on a study of mentally defective twins; ascertainment was from the New York State schools for mental defectives where a twin reporting system had been established in 1937. Among 645 twins so ascertained, 32 were mongols; they added several twin pairs to the study who had been referred to clinics. The zygosity of most of these twin pairs was diagnosed by blood group determinations and other objective methods (Table 5–6). To these data one can add the case reported by Dekaban, where one twin had a normal

Table 5–5. Distribution of Mongol Twins from Summary of Case Reports

		Dizygotic			
	Mono-zygotic	Both same sex	Different sex	Same sex but uncertainty about zygotic type	Total
One affected (discordant)	1	46	79	43	169
Both affected (concordant)	18	1	1	12	32
Total	19	47	80	55	201

Source: Penrose, L. S. & Smith, G. F. 1966. *Down's Anomaly* (Boston: Little, Brown and Company).

Table 5-6. Summary of Index Cases in Terms of Zygosity and Concordance

	Institutional series		Special cases		
	Concordant	Discordant	Concordant	Discordant	Total
Monozygotic	2	0	4	0	6
Dizygotic: Same sex	0	6	0	2	8
Opposite sex	0	14	0	1	15
Unknown zygosity	6	3	0	0	9
Total	8	23	4	3	38

Source: Allen, G. & Baroff, G. S. 1955. "Mongoloid twins and their siblings." *Acta Genet. Stat. Med.* 5: 294–326.

chromosomal complement and the other was a mongol with 48 chromosomes. A complex series of chromosomal errors has to be postulated to explain such an occurrence.

From the data presented, it appears fairly clear that among monozygotic twins there is about a 90–95 per cent concordance in mongols as compared to, at most, about 10 per cent concordance among dizygotic twins, even if one includes those series with uncertain diagnoses of zygosity. Probably the per cent concordance among dizygotes is much less than this. Such results are consistent with what would be expected from the chromosomal findings in mongolism.

Another feature of twin studies and their relation to mongolism was considered by Allen and Kallmann, who were interested in the frequency of twins among mongols. They determined this frequency among the institutionalized mongols and found it to be 1.95 per cent, which is what would be expected, but remains difficult to evaluate because of the selection of twins, mongols, etc. from institutions, and because of the excess mortality early in life for both twins and mongols. It would certainly be of interest to determine if there is an association between mongolism and twinning, particularly since maternal age affects the frequency of dizygotic twinning as it does mongolism. Thus, there may be an etiological relationship between these 2 conditions which should be investigated.

6:

The Association of Mongolism with Other Diseases

Mongolism and Leukemia

One of the more firmly established epidemiological facts about mongolism is the frequently confirmed observation that mongols have an increased risk of developing leukemia. The first case report appeared in 1930, followed by several other case reports which stimulated a statistical survey by Krivit and Good (Brewster & Cannon; Ingalls, 1947*a*; Merritt & Harris; Bernhard, Gore, & Kilby). They sent questionnaires to more than 300 medical centers in the United States asking about the simultaneous occurrence of these 2 diseases. The completed questionnaires of the 125 responding centers showed that 34 cases of mongolism simultaneous with leukemia had occurred in children under 5 years of age, during the period 1952–55. To determine whether or not this was a chance occurrence, the investigators estimated the number expected from previously determined incidence rates of mongolism and of leukemia. The details of the computations need not be presented here, but if chance alone were operating, 12.3 cases would be expected as a maximum. Since the observed number (34) was probably a minimal estimate because of obvious underreporting of such cases, the data were highly suggestive of a relationship between these 2 diseases.

Additional studies using the following 2 different study approaches were then conducted by several investigators: (1) the determination of the frequency of mongols among cases with leukemia, and (2) the determination of the frequency of, or mortality from, leukemia among mongols.

In each study approach, various types of comparison groups were selected, ranging from matched controls to estimated expected numbers of cases from national vital statistics data or conservative estimates of incidence rates of each of the diseases obtained from other investigations. It is unnecessary to describe these studies in detail; a summary of the studies describing the methods of selection, the comparison groups, and the results is presented in Tables 6–1 and 6–2. However, it should be noted that several of these studies were not directly concerned with this relationship per se, but the finding of this association was included in the general presentation of the study. For example, in studies on the survivorship of mongols, reports on the different causes of death of mongols which included leukemia, provided additional information on this relationship.

Table 6–1. Summary of Studies Showing Frequency of Mongols among Cases of Leukemia and a Comparison Group

		Leukemia cases			
				Mongols	
Investigator and year of report	Years of study	Methods of selection	Total number	Number	Per cent
Iverson (1960)	1946–57	Case records of patients under 15 years admitted to hospitals for first time with diagnosis of leukemia throughout Denmark.	273	5	1.8
Knox (1964)	1951–60	Leukemia in children with onset before 15th birthday in the North of England.	185	9	4.9
Stewart, Webb, & Hewitt (1958)	1953–55	Deaths from leukemia or cancer in children under 10 years of age in England and Wales.	677	17	2.5
Ager, Schuman, *et al.* (1965)	1953–57	Deaths under 5 years of age from leukemia in Minnesota.	124	9	7.2
Barber & Spiers (1964)	1953–60	Deaths from leukemia and other childhood cancers in England and Wales before age of 10 years.	1,795	49	2.7
Wald, Borges, *et al.* (1961)	1955–59	Leukemia deaths in Pennsylvania.	—	21	—
Miller (1963)	1958–61	Children with leukemia under 16 years of age in 12 medical groups in U.S. (white children).	459	6	1.3

Table 6–1 summarizes 7 studies reporting the frequency of mongols among cases of leukemia. In these studies the frequency of mongols ranged from 1.3 to 7.2 per cent as compared to 0.03 to 0.3 per cent among the comparison groups. The excess of mongols among leukemic children ranged from 6 to 100 times. Variations in the estimates of excess frequency of mongols are probably a result of differences in diagnostic criteria, as well as differences in methods of selection of comparison groups. Table 6–2 summarizes those studies on the frequency of leukemia among mongols, as compared to the observed frequency in a comparison group, or that expected on the basis of mortality experience. In general the frequency of leukemia is about 8 to 19 times greater among mongols than generally expected. Again, the variations no doubt reflect variation in the diagnostic criteria of leukemia and differences in the frequency of leukemia in the different geographical areas where the studies were

Table 6–1. Continued

Comparison group				
		Mongols		Degree of excess
Type	Total number	Number	Per cent	
Expected on basis of mongolism incidence of 1/600.	—	0.5	—	10
None.	—	—	—	—
a. Deaths from other cancers of childhood.	739	1	0.1	25
b. Live children matched for sex, age, locality.	1,416	0	0.0	—
Highest recorded incidence of mongolism.	—	—	0.3	21
a. Deaths from other cancers of childhood.	1,985	3	0.2	10–100
b. Live children matched for sex, age, locality.	3,778	1	0.03	—
Expected on basis of mongolism incidence of 1.5 per 1,000.	—	2	—	10
Neighborhood controls matched by age, birth order, family size, and race.	459	1 (expected based on incidence data) 0	0	6

Table 6–2. Summary of Studies Showing Frequency of Leukemia among Mongols and a Comparison Group or Expected Frequency Based on Mortality Experience

Investigator and year of report	Years of study	Mongols			
		Methods of selection	Total number	Leukemia	
				Number	Per cent
Merrit & Harris (1956)	1930–55	Cases diagnosed at Duke University Hospital.	255	4	1.6
Carter (1958)	1944–55	Survey of children who attended The Hospital for Sick Children in London to determine survivorship of mongols.	725	3	0.4
Holland, Doll, & Carter (1962)	1944–55	Children at The Hospital for Sick Children in London.	738	5	0.7
	1946–57	Children reported to Medical Officer of Health or to Mental Health Department of Middlesex County Council.	365	0	0
	1948–59	Patients diagnosed or admitted to one of 5 mental deficiency hospitals (survivorship).	930	2	0.2
	Total			7	
DeWolff (1964)	1945–61	Children examined at Hospital for Sick Children in Aarau (Switzerland).	134	5	3.7

conducted. However, it should be noted that in only 2 studies was an actual comparative group used, and in no study was an actual control group selected in a systematic random fashion (Holland, Doll, & Carter; DeWolff).

Turner (1962) carried out a detailed analysis of the relationship, using 2 different methods of study. First, he computed the age- sex-specific death rates from leukemia for Pennsylvania during the years 1955–60 and applied the rates to the estimated population of mongols. This determines the number of expected leukemia deaths among Pennsylvania mongols if the age- sex-specific leukemia death rates prevail. He then determined the number of leukemia deaths that had actually been observed in the mongol population and found an observed number of 19 such deaths, as compared to an expected number of 0.73, an excess of 26-fold (Table 6–3). After computing the age-sex-specific death rates from leukemia among the institutionalized mongols, he compared these with those of the general Pennsylvania population (Table 6–4). Since a selective bias may exist in a comparison of an institutionalized population with the general population, he went on to compare the leukemia incidence among institutionalized

Table 6–2. Continued

Comparison group				
		Leukemia		Degree of excess
Type	Total number	Number	Per cent	
None				
None				
Expected number of deaths from leukemia from national mortality rates.		0.19		
		0.06		
		0.14		
		0.39		18
Frequency of leukemia in hospital patients over 7-year period.	10,171	45	0.4	8–9

mongols with that among other mentally defective individuals who were also institutionalized. The leukemia death rate among mongols was 2.2 per 1,000 males and 1.7 for females, as compared with .08 per 1,000 males and 0.04 for females of other mental defectives. Table 6–5 contains the age- sex-specific observed number of leukemia deaths in the institutionalized mongol group, as compared to what would be expected if the death rates from leukemia in Pennsylvania had prevailed. The differences in observed and expected numbers are highly significant.

Of further interest is the observation that the increased risk of leukemia in the mongol population is present throughout life. Also, the increased incidence is not limited to any specific type of leukemia but involves the type appropriate to the age of the affected individual.

Another approach has been used to study this relationship. In addition to analyzing the frequency of mongolism among leukemic children, Miller (1963) examined the frequency of mongolism among the sibs of these leukemic children and compared this to the frequency among sibs of a group of matched controls. Of 1,000 sibs of the leukemic children, he observed 5 cases of mongolism as compared to

Table 6–3. Observed Versus Expected Number of Deaths Due to Leukemia in an Estimated Population of Pennsylvania Mongols, 1955–60

Age groups	Males: Number of mongols as of January 1, 1960	Males: Leukemia deaths: Annual rate (per 100,000)	Males: Leukemia deaths: Observed number	Males: Leukemia deaths: Expected number	Females: Number of mongols as of January 1, 1960	Females: Leukemia deaths: Annual rate (per 100,000)	Females: Leukemia deaths: Observed number	Females: Leukemia deaths: Expected number
1–4	313	5.9	2	0.111	313	3.6	3	0.068
5–9	337	5.9	1	0.119	298	2.4	1	0.043
10–14	255	1.9	3	0.090	245	1.8	3	0.026
15–19	198	2.4	2	0.070	182	1.2	0	0.013
20–24	140	1.4	0	0.050	135	2.4	0	0.019
25–29	106	4.8	1	0.037	91	0.9	0	0.005
30–34	100	1.9	1	0.025	73	1.8	1	0.008
35–39	79	3.1	0	0.028	52	2.6	1	0.008
Total	1,528		10	0.540	1,389		9	0.190

Note: Expected number computed by- Number mongols × Annual leukemia death rate × 6.
Source: Turner, J. H. 1962. "Mongoloid phenotype: Its incidence, etiology and association with leukemia and other neoplastic disease." Thesis, Sc.D. Hyg., University of Pittsburgh.

Table 6–4. Comparison of Age and Sex-Specific Leukemia Death Rates of the Institutionalized Mongol Population of Pennsylvania with Those of the General Pennsylvania Population

Age groups	Males: Average annual number mongols in institutions (1955–60)	Males: Leukemia deaths among mongols (1955–60): Number	Males: Leukemia deaths among mongols (1955–60): Average annual rate	Males: Annual leukemia death rate in general population	Females: Average annual number mongols in institutions (1955–60)	Females: Leukemia deaths among mongols (1955–60): Number	Females: Leukemia deaths among mongols (1955–60): Average annual rate	Females: Annual leukemia death rate in general population
0–4	1	41	406	5.9	1	34	490	3.6
5–9	1	100	167	5.9	1	75	222	2.4
10–14	2	102	327	1.9	2	68	490	1.8
15–19	1	83	201	2.4	0	55	000	1.2
20–24	0	55	000	1.4	0	36	000	2.4
25–29	1	57	292	4.8	0	38	000	0.9
30–34	1	48	347	1.9	1	36	463	1.8
35–39	0	35	000	3.1	1	27	617	2.6
40–	2	52	641	7.3–64.0	1	39	427	2.0–30.7
Total	9	573			7	408		

Note: Rates are per 100,000.

$$\text{Average annual death rate} = \frac{\text{Number leukemia deaths (1955–60)}}{\text{Average annual number mongols in institutions (1955–60)}} \times \frac{10^5}{6} = \text{deaths per 100,000 per year.}$$

Source: Turner, J. H. 1962. "The mongoloid phenotype: Its incidence, etiology and association with leukemia and other neoplastic disease." Thesis, Sc.D. Hyg., University of Pittsburgh.

1.4 expected from the frequency of mongolism in general and as compared to no mongols among the matched controls. Stark also studied this issue and reported finding 2 cases of acute childhood leukemia among 246 sibs of 91 mongolism cases, an observation which is consistent with Miller's observation.

There have also been several reports of newborn mongol infants who had, at the time of birth, conditions which resembled leukemia (Wegelius, Väänänen, & Koskela; Shunk & Lehman; Ross, Moloney, & Desforges; Engel, Hammond, *et al.*). However, follow-up of these children over a period of several years showed a remission of the blood picture. It is generally felt that these represent leukemoid reactions or as one investigator stated it "ineffective granulopoiesis masquerading as leukemia."

The relationship of mongolism to leukemia is of considerable interest in view of still other observations indicating that in mongols the nuclei of the polymorphonuclear cells have fewer lobes than normal

Table 6–5. Comparison by Age and Sex of Observed Versus Expected Number of Deaths Due to Leukemia and Other Neoplasms Occurring among the Institutionalized Population of Mongols, Pennsylvania, 1945–49

			Leukemia deaths			Deaths from other neoplasms		
Sex	Age groups	Number of mongols at risk	General population rate (per 1,000)	Observed number	Expected number	General population rate (per 1,000)	Observed number	Expected number
Males	0–4	250	0.059	1	0.0147	0.69	0	0.1725
	5–9	857	0.059	0	0.0505	0.37	0	0.3171
	10–14	1,380	0.019	2	0.0262	0.21	0	0.2898
	15–19	734	0.024	2	0.0176	0.54	0	0.3964
	20–24	399	0.014	0	0.0055	0.75	1	0.2992
	25–29	420	0.048	2	0.0201	1.04	0	0.4368
	30–34	374	0.019	1	0.0071	1.47	0	0.5498
	35–39	279	0.031	1	0.0086	2.60	1	0.7254
Total				9	0.1503		2	3.1870
Females	0–4	205	0.036	0	0.0074	0.50	0	0.1025
	5–9	647	0.024	2	0.0155	0.17	0	0.1553
	10–14	920	0.018	1	0.0166	0.32	0	0.1656
	15–19	490	0.012	1	0.0059	0.65	1	0.0589
	20–24	266	0.024	0	0.0064	0.98	2	0.0638
	25–29	280	0.009	0	0.0025	2.25	1	0.6300
	30–34	282	0.018	1	0.0051	4.52	1	1.2746
	35–39	219	0.026	1	0.0057	7.59	1	1.6622
Total				6	0.0651		6	4.1129

Note: Number of mongols at risk estimated from average annual population, 1945–49, × 15 years.

Source: Turner, J. H. 1962. "The mongoloid phenotype: Its incidence, etiology and association with leukemia and other neoplastic disease." Thesis, Sc.D. Hyg., University of Pittsburgh.

(Turpin & Bernyer; Shapiro; Lüers & Lüers; Mittwoch). It has also been pointed out that in mongols there is a shift to the left of the polymorphonuclear leucocytes and a decrease in the number of large lymphocytes. Mongols also have a decrease in the frequency of drumsticks (nuclear appendages) in their polymorphonuclear leucocytes.

Related to this is a finding in a great majority of cases of chronic granulocytic leukemia of what has been described as the Ph[1] (Philadelphia) chromosome. It is a specific abnormality in which one of chromosome pair 21 has lost approximately one-half of one of its arms; the cause or causes are unknown.

Explanations of the relationship of mongolism to leukemia are at present speculative. It has been suggested that a gene located on the trisomic chromosome pair 21 may control granulopoiesis. It has also been postulated that the relationship is indirect, that is, each disease may be a result of the same etiological agent. For example, radiation could produce nondisjunction and result in trisomy 21 and independently produce leukemia. Since the nondisjunction would have to take place prior to or immediately after conception, one would expect that mongols with leukemia would be most prevalent and perhaps even limited to the younger age groups. The only available data for evaluating this is Turner's which has been presented (Table 6–4) and indicates that the excess leukemia risk is present throughout life.

Pertinent to this hypothesis is the recently published report of an experiment in which 7, 12-dimethylbenz [a] anthracene (DMBA) in repeated doses produced trisomy of one group of chromosomes and leukemia in rats; this occurred in 10, or 43 per cent, of leukemic rats in 3 series of experiments (Sugiyama, Kurita, & Nishizuka). This confirmed a previous report of a similar experiment where in a different rat strain one case was produced by 7, 12-DMBA.

Another possible explanation is that individuals with chromosomal abnormalities have an increased susceptibility to environmental agents that produce leukemia. This hypothesis is compatible in a general way with that first suggested. If this hypothesis were true, one might suspect the relationship of other chromosomal abnormalities to leukemia. Recently, Fraumeni and Miller discussed various epidemiological aspects of leukemia and indicated that there is suggestive evidence of an increased risk of leukemia in other clinical syndromes with chromosomal abnormalities, such as the syndrome of Bloom and of Fanconi, although still other chromosomal disorders do not have an increased risk (Table 6–6).

Table 6–6. Congenital Cytogenetic Disorders and Leukemia–Lymphoma

Congenital disorder	Cytogenetic defect	Associated leukemia–lymphoma
Down's syndrome (mongolism)	Trisomy 21	Risk of leukemia known to be 20-fold or greater
Klinefelter's syndrome (seminiferous tubule dysgenesis)	XXY or mosaic	*Case reports* 1 acute myelogenous leukemia 1 chronic myelogenous leukemia 1 acute lymphocytic leukemia 2 reticulum cell sarcomas 1 acute undifferentiated leukemia
D-trisomy (Pätau's syndrome of multiple anomalies)	Trisomy in group 13–15	*Case reports* 1 congenital myeloblastic leukemia
Bloom's syndrome (low birth weight, stunted growth, sun-sensitive telangiectatic erythema of face)	Chromosome breakage and rearrangement of cultured blood cells	23 case reports 2 acute myelogenous leukemias 1 acute leukemia
Fanconi's syndrome (congenital pancytopenia with multiple anomalies)	Chromosome breakage and rearrangement of cultured blood cells	2 case reports with acute monocytic leukemia

Source: Fraumeni, J. F. & Miller, R. W. 1967. "Epidemiology of human leukemia: Recent observations." *J. Nat. Cancer Inst.* 38: 593–605.

Familial Aggregation of Mongolism and Leukemia

Another aspect of the relationship of mongolism with leukemia is the familial aggregation of these 2 conditions. There have been reports of the occurrence of leukemia among family members of mongols and of mongolism among family members of children with leukemia (Miller, Breg, *et al.*; Buckton, Harnden, *et al.*). The mortality experience of the parents of 1,620 mongol children was analyzed and compared with that expected from national death rates in England and Wales by Holland, Doll, and Carter. Their mortality from all causes was somewhat lower than expected; 3 deaths occurred from leukemia where 1.2 were expected and 57 deaths from other forms of cancer where 64 were expected. In a national cooperative study of leukemia in the U.S., Miller (1963) reported 5 cases of mongolism among 1,000 sibs of leukemia children, as compared to an expectancy of 1.4—a difference which was considered to be statistically significant. In contrast, Barber and Spiers did not observe such an excess frequency in their study of the sibs of 1,795 leukemia cases in England: 5.9 mongols were to be expected and 7 were actually observed.

Recently, Miller (1966) reviewed the relationship of malignancies to cytogenetic abnormalities as a basis for a conceptual etiological model. As part of this review, he summarized the case reports of the familial aggregation of mongolism and leukemia. Table 6–7, from his paper, summarizes the case reports for mongolism, as well as for other chromosomal abnormalities.

Table 6–7. Case Reports of Aggregation of Congenital Chromosomal Abnormalities and Leukemia in Families

Investigator and year of report	Type of leukemia	Chromosomal abnormality
	Sibships:	
Baikie, Court-Brown, *et al.* (1961)	Acute lymphocytic and acute myelogenous	XX/XXY mosaicism
Buckton, Harnden, *et al.* (1961)	Acute lymphocytic	Down's syndrome (15/21 translocation) in 3 sibs
Karhausen & Hutchison (1966)	Acute lymphocytic	Down's syndrome in 2 sibs
Conen, Erkman, & Laski (1966)	Acute stem cell	Down's syndrome in 2 sibs
	Families:	
Miller, Breg, *et al.* (1961)	Chronic lymphocytic (in father)	Son with XXXXY sex-chromosome complement; sister and niece with Down's syndrome (trisomy 21)
Heath & Moloney (1965)	Leukemia (5 cases)	Down's syndrome in 1 child

Source: Miller, R. W. 1966. "Relation between cancer and congenital defects in man." *New Eng. J. Med.* 275: 87–93.

It is difficult to evaluate these case reports of familial aggregation because it is impossible to determine the statistical significance of the reports. The 2 controlled studies have conflicting results (Barber & Spiers; Miller, 1966). However, even if one accepts Miller's results, it is clear that the degree of familial aggregation is small.

Mongolism and Thyroid Disease

For a long time there has been a great deal of interest and discussion on a possible relationship between thyroid disease and mongolism initiated by Benda and Bixby, who thought that mongolism was a pituitary disorder which caused secondary hypothyroidism. This view is not accepted today. Several investigators have performed a variety of tests of thyroid function on mongols, including determinations of protein-bound iodine, serum cholesterol, basal metabolism rates, and thyroid uptake of I–131; these have all been found to be normal. However, several investigators have reported an increase in the erythrocyte uptake of I–131 labelled triiodothyronine (Hayles, Hinrichs, & Tauxe; Saxema & Pryles). It isn't clear whether this is actually a reflection of differences in thyroid function or a secondary effect due to diminished serum albumin (Spinelli-Ressi & Bergonzi).

There have also been case reports in the literature on the frequency of hypothyroidism and hyperthyroidism among mongols; about 20 cases of hyperthyroidism and about 5 cases of hypothyroidism have been reported (Hayles, Hinrichs, & Tauxe; Jagiello & Taylor; Kay & Esselborn). It is completely impossible from these individual reports to determine whether there is a relationship between either hyperthyroidism or hypothyroidism and mongolism. The general impression is that the concurrence of these clinical diseases is not sufficiently frequent to warrant an inference of any relationship between them.

Thyroid Autoantibodies. Stimulated by finding an association of other types of chromosomal abnormalities with the presence of thyroid autoantibodies, in 1963 Mellon, Pay, and Green studied 35 cases of mongolism and found thyroid autoantibodies in 7, a contrast to finding none among the 35 matched controls. Of additional interest was their finding that 4 of the patients with antibodies had the more unusual types of chromosomal abnormalities associated with mongolism, such as mosaicism and translocations. There are 3 possible explanations for this association: (1) the chromosomal abnormality produced the thyroid antibodies; (2) thyroid antibodies produced the chromosomal abnormalities; or (3) both may be the result of the same etiological factor. To discriminate between these hypotheses, particularly the first from both the second and third, family studies were carried out by Fialkow, Uchida, Hecht, and Motulsky (Fialkow, 1966). Forty-four families with a mongol member were examined and compared with control families. The mongol families came from the Genetics Clinic of the University of Washington and from a private school for the mentally retarded. The control families were derived from outpatient clinics of the University of Washington Hospital or the Children's Orthopedic Hospital, which they were attending while a child was receiving well baby care, or because their child had hemophilia, muscular dystrophy, or another genetic disorder. Control families were matched with the mongol families for maternal age. The parents were interviewed and had their thyroid glands palpated. Nine (20 per cent) of 44 mothers of mongol patients had thyroid abnormalities, in contrast to 3 (7 per cent) of 44 control mothers. Two of 42 mongol fathers had clinical thyroid disease in contrast to none of the fathers of the control families. These results were of borderline statistical significance.

The study group was expanded in order to determine the presence of thyroid autoantibodies. The results expressed in terms of the per cent of mothers who had thyroid autoantibodies are presented in

Table 6–8. Thyroid Autoantibodies in Winnipeg and Seattle Females

Group	Number (and per cent) seropositive: Seattle families Number = 44	Number (and per cent) seropositive: Winnipeg families Number = 104	X^2	P value
Mothers of Down's patients	11 (25 per cent)	31 (30 per cent)	0.38	0.6
Control females	6 (13 per cent)	15 (14 per cent)	0.06	0.8
Total	17	45	0.30	0.6

Source: Fialkow, P. J. 1966. "Autoimmunity and chromosomal abberations." *Amer. J. Hum. Genet.* 18: 93–108.

Table 6–8. When the frequency of thyroid antibodies in these 2 groups was analyzed by maternal age, the mothers had a consistently higher frequency for all ages, except for the oldest (Table 6–9). No differences were observed between the fathers of the mongols and controls. It is still not clear whether the maternal antibodies antedated the birth of the child, for it is possible that the child with a chromosomal abnormality might stimulate the production of antibodies in the mother during pregnancy. Only a prospective study of pregnant women could answer this question directly. Evidence for this could be obtained by a study of the normal siblings of the mongol children. Such studies are now in progress.

A later report by Fialkow (1967) on a larger series indicates that the increase of these autoantibodies appears to be limited to mothers who were under 35 years of age when the mongol was born. They also appear to be more highly related to mongols of the non-trisomic types—mosaics and translocations. Engel in a later report found no particular relationship between antibodies and the chromosomal type of mongol. Other investigators have confirmed these findings (Dallaire & Flynn, 1967*b*; Burgio, Severi, *et al.*; Saxema & Pryles).

Fialkow (1966), in considering possible interpretations of these results, feels strongly that maternal thyroid autoantibodies directly or indirectly predispose to the child's chromosomal abnormalities. He points out that thyroxine may induce errors in chromosomal distribution in vitro. Another possibility is that a virus may lead to both autoimmunity and chromosomal abnormalities. Since these are attractive hypotheses, they should be tested by field epidemiological studies.

Table 6–9. Thyroid Autoantibodies in Mothers of Down's Syndrome Children Compared to Control Females

Age range (at time of testing)	Mothers of Down's patients: Number tested	Positive: Number	Positive: Per cent	Control females: Number tested	Positive: Number	Positive: Per cent	X^2	*P* value
20–32	52	14	27	52	2	4	8.9	<0.005
33–45	58	18	31	58	8	14	4.0	<0.05
46–60	38	10	26	38	11	29	0.066	>0.8
Total (20–60)	148	42	28	148	21	14	8.0	<0.005
Total in childbearing age (20–45)	110	32	29	110	10	9	13.0	<0.001

Note: A subject was counted as positive if the TRC titer was at least 1:9 or the IF titer was at least 1:10. X^2 calculated using Yate's correction for continuity.

Source: Fialkow, P. J. 1966. "Autoimmunity and chromosomal aberrations." *Amer. J. Hum. Genet.* 18:93–108.

Mongolism and Other Chromosomal Abnormalities

In the literature there have been 8 case reports of individuals who have both Klinefelter's and Down's syndromes (Benirschke, Brownhill, *et al.*; Ford, Jones, *et al.*; Harnden, Miller, & Penrose; Lanman, Sklarin, *et al.*; Lehmann & Forssman; MacLean, Mitchell, *et al.*; Wright, Day, *et al.*; Hustinx, Eberle, *et al.*). This has prompted the speculation that there may be a genetic predisposition to meiotic nondisjunction that produces the concurrence of both mongolism and Klinefelter's syndrome in the same individual.

Individual case reports of this dual syndrome are difficult to evaluate since the concurrence of both of these diseases may increase the chances of the patients receiving medical attention and subsequently being reported. Estimates have been made of the probability of this concurrence. Early estimates suggested that this concurrence would only occur in one of 560,000 total births. However, the estimate did not account for the fact that the frequency of each of these conditions increases with increasing maternal age. When this is taken into account, the estimated expected frequency of concurrence is one in 10,000 total births (Hamerton, Jagiello, & Kirman).

Clearly the best approach to clarify this question would be to survey a group of mongol children and determine the frequency of Klinefelter's syndrome. An approximation to this type of survey was conducted by Mikkelsen and Frøland, who carried out a sex chromatin survey of 1,162 mongol patients in Danish institutions. The frequency of sex chromatin abnormalities in this group did not differ from that previously observed in normal newborn children.

From the latter it would appear that there is no unusual concordance of these 2 conditions. However, it would be of interest to have a few additional surveys similar to that conducted by Mikkelsen and Frøland to definitely rule out the possibility of concurrence.

Mongolism and Other Diseases

Over the past several years, reports have appeared on a series of cases suggesting an association of Hirschsprung's disease with mongolism. These have been recently summarized by Passarge (Table 6–10). Of 1,163 cases of Hirschsprung's disease, 2.05 per cent, or 24 cases of mongolism have been observed. Whether this frequency is greater than that expected by chance is difficult to determine. Further study with more adequate controls is necessary for a more definitive assessment.

There is no need to document the well-known association of mongolism with other types of congenital malformations. These are well known and have been extensively reviewed most recently by Penrose and Smith. The strongest association is with congenital heart disease where 40–60 per cent of mongols in the various reports have been found to have one or more forms of congenital heart disease.

Table 6–10. Frequency of Down's Syndrome in Patients with Hirschsprung's Disease

Investigator and year of report	Patients with Down's syndrome	Total
Althoff (1962)	1	68
Bodian & Carter (1963)	3	207
Madsen (1964)	1	157
Gordon, Torrington, *et al.* (1966)	1	56
Emanuel, Padorr, & Swenson (1965)	3	287
Hofmann & Rehbein (1966)	5	222
Graivier & Sieber (1966)	3	84
Hays & Norris (1956)	1	19
Passarge (1967)	6	63
Total	24 (2.05 per cent)	1,163

Source: Passarge, E. 1967. "The genetics of Hirschsprung's disease: Evidence for heterogeneous etiology and a study of sixty-three families." *New Eng. J. Med.* 276: 138–43.

7:

Selected Characteristics of Mongols Including Mortality Experience

It is beyond the scope of a review on the epidemiology of mongolism to consider in complete detail the characteristics of mongols, particularly since several excellent and detailed reviews of this subject have been recently published, including both the clinical and biochemical characteristics (Penrose & Smith; Stern). However, it is recognized that certain characteristics can be pertinent to etiological hypotheses or might lead to epidemiological studies. An integral part of the entire spectrum of characteristics is the association of mongolism and other diseases, reviewed in Chapter 6, which also includes a consideration of physical or biochemical characteristics relevant to specific clinical diseases. This chapter will be concerned with blood groups, a variety of biochemical studies, and mortality experience.

Blood Groups

There was an early interest in the blood group distribution of mongols stimulated by the original hypothesis of Langdon-Down of a genetic relationship between mongolism and Mongolian populations (Penrose, 1932). Studies at the time indicated that the blood group distributions of mongols were similar to those of control groups living in the same countries.

As interest developed in the possible influence of blood group incompatibilities in fetal and neonatal mortality, investigators explored the possible role of this factor in mongolism, with negative results

(Lang-Brown, Lawler, & Penrose; Hackel). However, the cytogenetic findings in turn stimulated interest in the study of blood groups and in the different types of hemoglobins in an attempt to determine whether the genetic loci of these blood groups are on the extra mongol chromosome.

Biochemical Studies

A variety of biochemical studies on mongols have been performed by many different investigators. Earlier these studies were etiologically oriented and reflected the interest of the investigators in the possible influence of hormonal abnormalities. Since the finding of the chromosomal abnormality, geneticists have been interested in determining whether a genetic locus that controls enzyme formation or any other biochemical parameter is located on the extra chromosome. Such relationships, however, are not particularly relevant to epidemiological studies. In view of the recent reviews on this subject and conforming to the primary purpose of this book we considered it sufficient to present the results of these biochemical studies in summary form (Table 7–1).

A review of this summary quite clearly reveals a high degree of variability in findings by the different observers. Although initially this variability is quite puzzling, closer scrutiny of the reports provides some possible explanations: (1) there is variability in the methods used by the different investigators; (2) in many instances, the number of mongols tested is small and may not be sufficient to permit detecting a substantial difference between mongols and controls, if in fact a difference does exist; (3) some of the biochemical parameters are influenced by age and, in many of the studies, age differences were not accounted for in the comparisons of mongols with controls; (4) of interest is the observation that in many of the reports a certain proportion of the mongols differed from the normals; (5) some of these observed differences are related to the type of mongolism—for example, trisomic mongols have been reported to have higher levels of several enzymes than translocation mongols; this may reflect a genetic overdose resulting from the additional chromosome (Rosner, Ong, *et al.*, 1965*a*); (6) most of the studies were performed on institutionalized mongols. When institutionalized and noninstitutionalized mongols have been studied, it has been observed that noninstitutionalized mongols are similar to controls but the institutionalized group differs from both. It is quite possible that institutionalization with its at-

Table 7–1. Summary of Findings of Studies of Biochemical Characteristics of Mongols

Biochemical determination	Findings			
Serum calcium	Normal (4–6,58)			Low (1–3)
Serum inorganic phosphate	Normal (1,4–5)		Slight increase (2)	
Serum sodium, potassium, chloride, bicarbonate	Normal (1,5,7)			
Serum magnesium			Elevated (8)	
Serum proteins:				
1) Total	Normal (1,9–10,53)			
2) Albumin	Normal (11,53,55)			Decreased (1,9–10)
3) Gamma globulin	Normal (11) (in noninstitutional cases)	Different structure (54,56)	Increased (1,9–11,52,55)	
4) Alpha and beta globulins	Normal (10,53)			
5) Haptoglobins	Normal (12)			
6) Transferrins	Normal (12)			
Blood sugar	Normal (1,5,13,53)			Decreased (14)
Glucose tolerance curves		Abnormal (4–5,14–16)		
Insulin tolerance test		Abnormal (14)		
Cholesterol	Normal (1,5,17,53)		Increased (17–18)	
Phospholipids			Increased (17)	
Lipoproteins	Normal (21)	Abnormal pattern (19)	Increased (18,20)	
Amino acids:				
1) Tryptophane metabolism	Normal (27)	Abnormal (22–26)		
2) Serotonic activity in blood				Lowered (28)
3) Beta aminoisobutyric acid in urine	Normal (31,53,59)		Increased (29–30)	
4) Taurine excretion				Lower (59)
5) Serum amino acids	Normal (59)			
Adreno-cortical hormones	Normal (33–35,53)	Deficiency (5,32,57)		
Enzymes:				
1) Leukocyte alkaline phosphatase			Increased (36–39,58)	
2) Serum phosphatase, and aromatic esterase	Normal (1–2,53)			
3) Serum pseudocholinesterase				Decreased (3,40)
4) Galactose-1-phosphate-uridyl-transferase in leukocytes			Increased (41–44,58)	

Table 7–1. Continued

Biochemical determination	Findings	
5) Galactose-1-phosphate-uridyl-transferase in red blood cells	Normal (45)	Increased (58)
6) G-6-P-dehydrogenase	Normal (43)	Increased (44,58)
7) Erythrocyte-galactokinase		Elevated (45–46)
8) Erythrocyte-phosphohexokinase		Increased (47)
Serum uric acid	Normal (1,58)	Increased (48–51)

Source:

1. Sobel, Strazzula, *et al.*
2. Stern & Lewis (1958)
3. Berg & Stern
4. Bixby (1939)
5. Benda (1960)
6. Maas
7. Bixby (1940)
8. Stern & Lewis (1959–60)
9. Donner
10. Stern & Lewis (1957*a*)
11. Pritham, Appleton, & Fluck
12. Hutton & Smith
13. Bixby & Benda
14. Runge
15. Brousseau & Brainerd
16. O'Leary
17. Stern & Lewis (1957*b*)
18. Simon, Ludwig, *et al.*
19. Stern & Lewis (1959)
20. Nelson
21. Benda & Mann
22. O'Brien & Groshek
23. Gershoff, Hegsted, & Trulson
24. Jérôme, Lejeune, & Turpin
25. Jérôme
26. O'Brien, Zarins, & Jensen
27. McCoy & Chung
28. Rosner, Ong, *et al.* (1965*b*)
29. Lundin & Gustavson
30. Wright & Fink
31. Perry, Shaw, & Walker
32. Sandrucci & Piccotti
33. Dutton
34. O'Sullivan, Reddy, & Farrell
35. Rundle, Dutton, & Gibson
36. Alter, Lee, *et al.*
37. Trubowitz, Kirman, & Masek
38. King, Gillis, & Baikie
39. Lennox, White, & Campbell
40. Stern & Lewis (1962)
41. Brandt
42. Brandt, Frøland, *et al.*
43. Hsia, Inouye, *et al.*
44. Mellman, Oski, *et al.*
45. Krone, Wolf, *et al.*
46. Donnell, Ng, *et al.*
47. Baikie, Loder, *et al.*
48. Fuller, Luce, & Mertz
49. Mertz, Fuller, & Concon
50. Chapman & Stern
51. Goodman, Lofland, & Thomas
52. Yokoyama
53. Pozsonyi & Gibson
54. Fluck
55. Skanse & Laurell
56. Appleton, Haak, *et al.*
57. Reiss, Wakoh, *et al.*
58. Rosner, Ong, *et al.* (1965*a*)
59. King, Goodman, & Thomas

tendant dietary changes and environment may affect the endocrine system which in turn may affect various biochemical measurements. This may be a major reason for many of the reported differences; this possible bias needs further investigation.

Australia Antigen. Recently Blumberg, Gerstley, Hungerford, London, and Sutnick reported finding a new isoantigen in the sera of mongol patients; because it was found in an Australian aborigine it has been given the name "Australia Antigen." The frequency of this antigen in different groups as reported by the authors is presented in Table 7–2. This finding is of particular interest because it has also been found in patients with hepatitis and leukemia. The antigen may thus reflect some underlying common denominator in these diseases, perhaps a viral infection, since some of these diseases have been shown to have a relationship with each other. It is hoped that the additional research on this antigen now in progress will shed some further light on this matter.

Variability of Mongols

In reviewing the literature on the characteristics of mongols, one is struck by the large degree of variability among mongols. Levinson,

Table 7–2. Distribution of Australia Antigen in Patients and U.S. Normals

Disease	Number tested	Positive	
		Number	Per cent
A-beta-lipoproteinemia	6	0	0.0
Amyotrophic lateral sclerosis	15	0	0.0
Anemia, various	26	0	0.0
Arthritis	70	0	0.0
Cancer, other than leukemias	95	0	0.0
Diabetes	303	0	0.0
Down's syndrome (mongolism)	84	25	29.8
Fanconi's anemia (hypoplasia bone marrow)	2	1	—
Hemophilia	60	3	5.0
Hepatitis, virus	48	5	10.4
Hodgkin's disease	12	1	8.3
Hypercholesterolemia	17	0	0.0
Leukemia and related diseases	177	16	9.0
Lupus erythematosus	69	0	0.0
Multiple myeloma and macroglobulinemia	95	1	1.1
Myasthenia gravis	11	0	0.0
Polycythemia vera	82	0	0.0
Rheumatic fever	124	0	0.0
Tangier disease	3	0	0.0
Thalassemia	84	2	2.4
U.S. normal population	1,524	0	0.0
White 917			
Negro 607			
Total	2,907	54	

Source: Blumberg, B. S., Gerstley, B. J. S., Hungerford, D. A., London, W. T., & Sutnick, A. I. 1967. "A serum antigen (Australia Antigen) in Down's syndrome, leukemia and hepatitis." *Ann. Int. Med.* 66: 924–31.

Friedman, and Stamps in 1955 stated, "most physicians seem to believe that mongolism not only has a constant clinical picture with definite physical and developmental characteristics but that there can be no question of degree of mongolism or transitional forms between classical mongolism and the normal state. . . . The data presented in this paper . . . shows that there is a wide range of variability in every single physical and developmental characteristic of mongoloids as well as in the sum total of such characteristics in each individual case."

More recently, Goodman, Lofland, and Thomas have stated:

> the theoretical considerations included provide a basis for a genetic interpretation of a fact long known from the study of mongoloids, namely, that no stigma or sign is common to all mongoloids and few mongoloids have all of the stigmata associated with mongolism. The concept that any parameter of biochemical significance in a given disease will be common to all individuals with the disease has been most useful in diseases due to single etiologic agents such as cystic fibrosis or tuberculosis. However, this concept has tended to impede progress in diseases of complex etiology. Many current papers refer to "the mongoloid"

child when in most cases, the abnormality is found in only a fraction of the mongoloid children studied.

One can, as Goodman, Lofland, and Thomas do, relate the observed variability to the differences in the genetic content of the extra chromosome. However, it is also possible that the variability reflects differential effects of different etiological agents on the genetic constitution. From an epidemiological viewpoint, it would be extremely valuable to determine the relationship of more homogeneous subgroups of mongols to factors of epidemiological interest, such as maternal age. This will be discussed further in Chapter 8.

Mortality Experience

Several studies on the mortality experience of mongols have been reported. Data from these reports have been collated and summarized in the form of a life table showing the per cent of mongols who have survived to a given age (Table 7–3). The life table data in general confirm the clinical impression that there has been an improvement in the mortality experience of mongols as a result of the use of antibiotics in the treatment of respiratory infections in infancy and childhood. At the present time, it appears that about 25–30 per cent of mongols die during the first year of life and about 50 per cent during the first 5 years.

The most recent study of mortality experience was reported by Forssman and Akesson (1965) for 1,263 patients enrolled in Swedish institutions for the mentally retarded. The mortality experience for mongols of all ages was 6 per cent higher than that of the general population. No differences were noted between the sexes, a difference

Table 7–3. Summary of Studies of Survivorship Experience of Mongols by Number of Years after Birth

	Investigator and year of report, years of study, and number of cases				
Number of years after birth	Carter (1958) 1944–55 698	Record & Smith (1955) 1942–52 252	Lunn (1959) 1953–58 116	Collmann & Stoller (1963*b*) 1948–57 729	Turner (1963) 1945–59 8,002
			Per cent survivors		
1	46.9	45.6	72.3	68.9	55.0
2	43.3	43.3	60.5	57.9	—
3	42.1	41.7	—	54.0	—
4	40.5	41.3	—	51.4	—
5	39.6	40.3	—	49.4	45.9
10	36.8	—	—	46.2	39.7

Table 7–4. Mortality in 1,236 Patients with Down's Syndrome, by Age

Age groups	Number of persons	Number of deaths	*R*	*P*	*R/P*
1–4	69	11	495	554	0.89
5–9	235	18	1,803	1,880	0.96
10–14	323	16	2,552	2,624	0.97
15–19	174	13	1,279	1,339	0.96
20–24	99	10	743	801	0.93
25–29	98	8	752	792	0.95
30–39	163	16	1,240	1,313	0.94
40–49	69	16	460	538	0.86
50–	33	18	166	236	0.70
Total	1,263	126	9,490	10,077	0.94

Note: *R* = Number of years persons studied survived during period of observation. *P* = Number of years equal number of persons same age in normal population could be expected to survive during same period.

Source: Forssman, H. & Akesson, H. O. 1965. "Mortality in patients with Down's syndrome." *J. Ment. Defic. Res.* 9:146–49.

reported earlier by Penrose (1949), Record and Smith, and Collmann and Stoller (1963*b*). These results for the different ages are presented in Table 7–4. In view of the relatively small numbers in some age groups, some of the variability may represent sampling fluctuation.

Causes of death were reported by Record and Smith, Carter, and Øster, Mikkelsen, and Nielsen. The distribution of these causes as compared to those expected on the basis of general mortality experience was reported by Øster, Mikkelsen, and Nielsen for 524 mongols who died during the 10-year period, 1949–59 (Table 7–5). The most frequent causes of death were respiratory and other infectious diseases, followed by congenital heart disease, a finding consistent with observations by other investigators.

Table 7–5. Observed and Expected Number of Deaths among Mongols by Cause of Death

Cause of death	Number of deaths: Observed	Number of deaths: Expected	Observed/Expected
Infectious diseases, excluding tuberculosis	5	0.097	52
Tuberculosis	—	0.128	—
Malignant conditions	4	1.180	3
Accidents, poisoning, and violence	2	1.136	2
Suicide	—	0.685	—
Respiratory disease	37	0.299	124
Cardiac disease	13	1.213	11
Senile disease and apoplexy	3	0.363	8
Other causes	9	2.640	3

Note: Malignant conditions include 2 cases of leukemia.

Source: Øster, J., Mikkelsen, M., & Nielsen, A. 1964. "The mortality and causes of death in patients with Down's syndrome (mongolism)," in: *Proc. International Copenhagen Congress on the Scientific Study of Mental Retardation*, vol. 1, pp. 231–35.

8:

Etiological Hypotheses and Suggested Epidemiological Research

In the course of presenting each of the different epidemiological aspects of mongolism, consideration has been given to the etiological inferences that can be derived from the data under discussion, and throughout the review, specific needs for additional epidemiological research have also been indicated. It seems desirable, therefore, at this point to consolidate the different etiological hypotheses and discuss them in a unified manner. It also seems appropriate to include a broad description of additional epidemiological studies which would fill some of the gaps in our knowledge on mongolism or which would provide some leads for tests of various etiological hypotheses.

Etiological Hypotheses

The most complete formulation of a set of etiological hypotheses for mongolism has been developed and presented in a series of papers by Penrose and summarized in Penrose and Smith's "Down's Anomaly." A brief review of his formulation will provide a useful framework for the present discussion. Penrose groups the causes according to their dependence on maternal age as follows:

(1) Independent of mother's age

- a. Secondary nondisjunction
- b. Translocation or other anomaly of the critical chromosome in a parent
- c. Genes which tend to produce nondisjunction
- d. Environmental influences

(2) Dependent on mother's age
    a. Oocyte deterioration
    b. Risks for very young mothers

Each of the subcategories will be discussed briefly.

(1) *a.* Secondary nondisjunction. This occurs when trisomy is present in the mother. As is clear from the data presented in Chapter 5, this is a rare occurrence. However, secondary nondisjunction also occurs if the mother is a mosaic mongol and the gonads (ovary and testes) contain the trisomic cells. Penrose indicates that only a few such cases have been reported. Nevertheless, he estimates that the frequency of mongolism caused by trisomic mothers is about 10 per cent and by trisomic fathers, 1 per cent; these are based on the frequency of dermatoglyphic microsymptoms among parents of mongols. One must, however, view this estimate with caution for the acceptance of dermatoglyphic patterns as indicating microsymptoms of mongolism is not universal; it is, at best, an indirect measure of mosaicism. There is a real need to determine the frequency of mosaic gonads among parents of mongols as an estimate of the contribution of such mosaicism to the frequency of mongolism. Some possible techniques for this purpose have recently been reported (Jagiello, Karnicki, & Ryan).

b. Inherited translocation or other anomaly of the critical chromosome. Inherited translocation is discussed in Chapter 5. There are several additional abnormalities that occur during meiosis; they result from inversions in chromosomes or from other abnormalities in chromosome morphology. The tendency of satellited chromosomes to associate has been suggested as an explanation for the increase in the frequency of aberrations involving those chromosomes.

c. Genes tending to produce nondisjunction. It has been hypothesized from analogies in drosophila that genes can produce nondisjunction. Penrose estimated that at most about 5 to 10 per cent of mongols can be attributed to this mechanism. However, the review of the data on consanguinity and familial aggregation presented in Chapter 5 does not provide any definitive evidence for genetic influences on nondisjunction.

d. Environmental influences. Many environmental influences have been hypothesized as causing nondisjunction. Maternal illness, radiation exposure, viruses, endocrine factors, and others, all of which have been studied, and discussed in selected sections of this review. It is clear that even though evidence is now available on the influence of many of these factors, confirmation by additional studies is in order.

(2) *a.* Oocyte deterioration. Penrose has postulated that the increasing incidence of mongolism with increasing maternal age is a result of progressive deterioration of the oocyte by accidental occurrences, reflecting the natural aging of the nucleus of the ovum. A discussion of this hypothesis is presented in Chapter 2.

b. Risks for very young mothers. There is apparently a suggestion of a slight increase in the risk for mongolism among very young mothers (15 to 29 years of age); this may actually reflect the possible increased risk among first-born reported by some investigators. The latter relationship has been reviewed in Chapter 2, and it is doubtful that there is an excess risk among young mothers.

Penrose has estimated the proportion of mongols that can be attributed to each of these etiological categories, noting that they are very rough estimates (Table 8–1).

Although Penrose's classification of possible causes is generally useful, it is not clear what purpose is served by the initial classification of causes according to maternal age dependency status. In fact, Penrose's estimates of the proportion of mongols in each category is influenced by his estimate of the proportions assigned to maternal age categories. As has already been pointed out (Chapter 2), this propor-

Table 8–1. Partition of Causes of Down's Syndrome

Relationship with maternal age	Cause	Possible proportion in an unselected group (per cent)
	Class A	
Independent of mother's age	(1) Inevitable nondisjunction (parent partly or wholly trisomic).	10
	(2) Abnormality in chromosome pairing (inherited translocation, inversion or other anomaly of the critical G-chromosome).	10
	(3) Abnormal meiosis or mitosis (specific genes which cause nondisjunction).	10
	(4) Environmental disturbance of cell division (infection, poison, radiation).	10
	Class B	
Dependent upon mother's age	Nondisjunction during oogenesis (deterioration of meiotic cell-division mechanism).	60

Source: Penrose, L. S. & Smith, G. F. 1966. *Down's Anomaly* (Boston: Little, Brown, and Company).

tion is influenced to some extent by the maternal age distribution of live births.

It would be more useful to classify the mongols according to type: trisomy, translocation, and mosaic. For each type, one can then evaluate specific genetic and environmental influences, since one would expect that the individual types may well have different causes. For example, in the case of translocation, studies have indicated that 25 per cent are inherited from a carrier (Chapter 5). Operationally, any effort to elucidate other genetic or environmental causes of translocations must be limited to the so-called sporadic types. In fact, one can recommend a general principle that any search for etiological factors should focus on the specific chromosomal types of mongolism.

If the etiological factors are considered in terms of the specific types of mongolism, the maternal age relationship then becomes one of the epidemiological facts that must be explained by one or more etiological theories. The distinction between this mode of thinking and Penrose's is a subtle one, but, operationally it appears as a more reasonable approach for further research.

The etiological hypotheses that have been presented by several investigators are based on the following etiological model *A*, assuming there are multiple etiological factors:

ETIOLOGICAL MODEL A

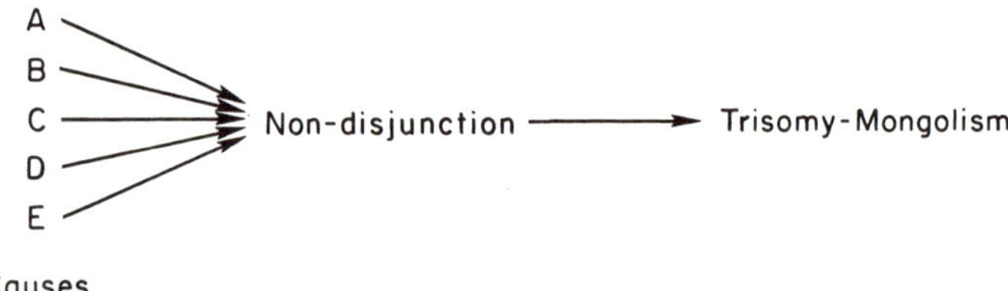

One of the problems generally encountered in the study of diseases involving multiple etiological factors is the difficulty in obtaining a strong relationship with any one particular factor. Thus, it is quite possible that radiation exposure of the mother may be of etiological significance, but the results of studies will continue to be unimpressive since it may well be only one among many possible factors. It would be helpful in this situation if the disease could be classified according to another set of parameters.

In searching for another dimension, we have been impressed by several reports suggesting that mongolism is perhaps not as homogeneous a clinical entity as is usually assumed. We note for instance that not all, but about 35 per cent of mongols, have different types of congenital heart disease, and less frequently they have other congenital malformations. In addition, many variations in their physical signs have been noted (Levinson, Friedman, & Stamps).

Perhaps this variability reflects the influence of different etiological agents. Thus, it is conceivable that agent *A* produces trisomy and another genetic change which results in mongolism with congenital heart disease, while agent *B* produces trisomy and still another type of malformation associated with mongolism. This can be figuratively shown in the following model *B*. Of course, combinations of causes and mechanisms must also be considered as a possibility. Rohde has also pointed out this heterogeneity in mongolism, as well as in the other trisomic syndromes, but has explained it on a strictly genetic basis.

ETIOLOGICAL MODEL B

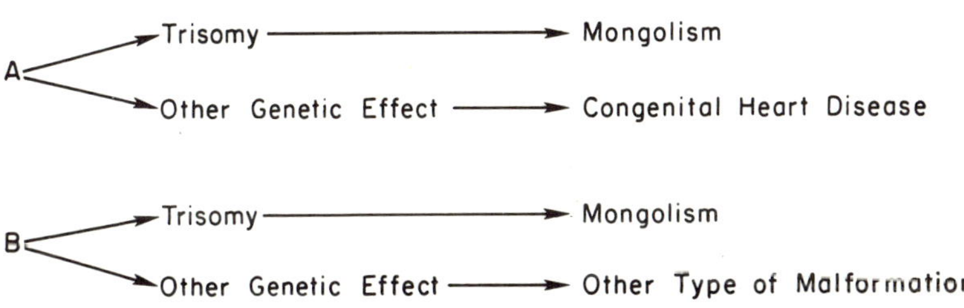

With model *B* in mind in searching for etiological agents, it would appear extremely profitable to think in terms of homogeneous groups of mongols. Unfortunately, this requires large scale studies simultaneously conducted in several cities in order to obtain the necessary number of cases in the different homogeneous subgroups.

Suggested Epidemiological Research

At appropriate points in this review, specific research needs have been briefly indicated. They usually recommended further study of specific relationships. It did not appear necessary to collate and summarize these suggestions; rather, we thought it would be more profitable to suggest several large-scale research projects that, from an epidemiological viewpoint, deserve a high priority.

Since geographical and ethnic differences in incidence may provide clues to etiology, it would be beneficial to select as areas of study, several large cities in the United States, India, Africa, Yugoslavia, and Israel, countries where there is suggestive evidence of wide differences in incidence rates. In each city, for a number of years, all newborns should be clinically evaluated for mongolism and have their chromosomes examined, using uniform criteria. Samples of normal newborns should also have chromosomal analyses. It would also be profitable to include chromosomal studies of all or, of a sample, of abortions in these cities. A collaborative study would provide estimates of incidence rates of clinical mongolism and of trisomy conception. The comparisons of such incidence rates in these areas would be very revealing.

It would be desirable to test practically all of the known or postulated associations with mongolism, and at the same time to determine if there are any interactions between these factors, i.e., is each one independently associated with mongolism or is there an association with only a few? To conduct such a study, several large cities would have to be selected and an ascertainment of all mongols carried out; control groups would also have to be selected and included in the study. The mongols should be clinically examined and their chromosomes studied.

The characteristics of the parents of the mongols would be determined by an interview and clinical and laboratory examination. Information obtained from the mother should include history of radiation exposure, reproductive performance, history of various diseases, determination of thyroid antibody titers, the usual demographic data on ethnic background, lifetime residential, marital, and menstrual histories, etc. Similar types of information should be obtained from the father. The study should be as all-encompassing as possible in an attempt to confirm suggested existing relationships and to elucidate new ones. Several types of interesting and no doubt profitable comparisons could be made. For example, a comparison of the characteristics of trisomic mongols born to older mothers with those born to younger mothers, as well as of the characteristics of their parents, might provide clues clarifying the maternal age effect in mongolism. One would also be able to compare the various characteristics of homogeneous subgroups of mongols. For example, do mongols with congenital heart disease show a greater degree of association with maternal age at birth than those without congenital heart disease? Many interesting questions with direct relevance to etiological hypotheses can be raised and answered by such a study. However, it should be realized that this type of study would require a collaborative effort in several very large cities to insure a sufficient number of mongols in each subgroup.

In addition to these rather large-scale studies, one should not overlook the potentially profitable smaller studies which are concerned with a specific, limited issue. For example, it would be interesting to determine if meiotic nondisjunction in the ovary increases in frequency with age. This can now be studied, using the techniques developed by Jagiello, Karnicki, and Ryan. It would also be of interest to compare the distribution of maternal age at birth of mongols with heart disease and mongols with leukemia, as well as with those having other types of malformations. The characteristics of the parents of a group of sporadic translocations should be studied and compared with an adequate control group; this could include histories of radiation and drug exposure, occupational history, etc.

It is strikingly evident from this review of the epidemiology of mongolism that the present is a propitious time for embarking upon a major research program of broad scope in an effort to determine the etiological factors in mongolism that will provide a basis for developing preventive programs.

References

AGER, E. A., SCHUMAN, L. M., WALLACE, H. M., ROSENFIELD, A. B., and GULLEN, W. H. 1965. "An epidemiological study of childhood leukemia." *J. Chronic Dis.* 18: 113–32.

ÅKESSON, H. O. and FORSSMAN, H. 1966. " A study of maternal age in Down's syndrome." *Ann. Hum. Genet.* 29: 271–76.

ALLEN, G. and BAROFF, G. S. 1955. "Mongoloid twins and their siblings." *Acta Genet. Stat. Med.* 5: 294–326.

ALLEN, G. and KALLMANN, F. J. 1955. "Mongolism in twin sibships." *Amer. J. Hum. Genet.* 7: 385–93.

ALLISON, A. C. 1968. "Genetics and infectious disease," in: *Haldane and Modern Biology,* ed. K. R. DRONAMRAJU, pp. 179–201. Baltimore: The Johns Hopkins Press.

ALLISON, A. C. and PATON, G. R. 1966. "Chromosomal abnormalities in human diploid cells infected with mycoplasma and their possible relevance to the aetiology of Down's syndrome (mongolism)." *Lancet* 2: 1229–30.

ALTER, A. A., LEE, S. L., POURFAR, M., and DOBKIN, G. 1962. "Leukocyte alkaline phosphatase in mongolism: A possible chromosome marker." *J. Clin. Invest.* 41: 1341.

ALTHOFF , W. 1962. "Zur genetik der Hirschsprungschen krankheit." *Ztschr. Menschl. Vererb. Konstitutionslehre* 36: 314–40.

APPLETON, M. D., HAAB, W., HART, M. I., and NEARY, J. 1966–67. "Physical studies of mongoloid serum gamma-globulins." *Amer. J. Ment. Defic.* 71: 465–71.

ATKINS, L., O'SULLIVAN, M. A., PRYLES, C. V., and FLORY, D. A. 1962. "Mongolism in three siblings with 46 chromosomes." *New Eng. J. Med.* 266: 631–35.

AULA, P. and HJELT, L. 1964. "Cytogenetics in mongolism: A review of literature and personal investigation." *Ann. Paed. Fenn.* 10: 13–23.

AUSTIN, C. R. 1967. "Chromosome deterioration in ageing eggs of the rabbit." *Nature* 213: 1018–19.

BABBOTT, J. G. and INGALLS, T. 1962. "Field studies of selected congenital malformations occurring in Pennsylvania." *Amer. J. Public Health* 52: 2009–17.

BAIKIE, A. G., COURT-BROWN, W. M., BUCKTON, K. E., and HARNDEN, D. G. 1961. "Two cases of leukaemia and a case of sex-chromosome abnormality in the same sibship." *Lancet* 2: 1003–04.

BAIKIE, A. G., LODER, P. B., DEGRUCHY, G. C., and PITT, D. B. 1965. "Phosphohexokinase activity of erythrocytes in mongolism: Another possible marker for chromosome 21." *Lancet* 1: 412–14.

BAILAR, J. C. III and GURIAN, J. 1965. "Congenital malformations and season of birth: A brief review." *Eugen. Quart.* 12: 146–53.

BARBER, R. and SPIERS, P. 1964. "Oxford survey of childhood cancers: Progress report II." *Monthly Bull. Minst. Health* 23: 46–52.

BEIDLEMAN, B. 1945. "Mongolism: A selective review. Including an analysis of forty-two cases from the records of the Boston Lying-In Hospital." *Amer. J. Ment. Defic.* 50: 35–53.

BENDA, C. E. 1946. *Mongolism and Cretinism.* New York: Grune and Stratton.

———. 1960. *The Child with Mongolism (Congenital Acromicria).* New York, London: Grune and Stratton.

BENDA, C. E. and BIXBY, E. M. 1939. "Function of the thyroid and the pituitary in mongolism: With a report on the blood groups of American mongoloid defectives and comments on the determination of cholesterol." *Amer. J. Dis. Child.* 58: 1240–55.

BENDA, C. E. and MANN, G. V. 1955. "The serum cholesterol and lipoprotein levels in mongolism." *J. Pediat.* 46: 49–53.

BENIRSCHKE, K., BROWNHILL, L., HOEFNAGEL, D., and ALLEN, F. H., Jr. 1962. "Langdon-Down anomaly (mongolism) with 21/21 translocation and Klinefelter's syndrome in the same sibship." *Cytogenetics* 1: 75–89.

BEOLCHINI, P. E., BARIATTI, A. B., and MORGANTI, G. 1962. "Indagini genetico-statistiche sulle fratrie di 432 soggetti mongoloidi." *Acta Genet. Med. Gemell.* 11: 430–49.

BERG, J. M.: Discussion in: FORSSMAN, H. and ÅKESSON, H. O. 1967. "Consanguineous marriages and mongolism." Ciba Foundation Study Group No. 25, *Mongolism,* pp. 23–34. Boston: Little, Brown and Company.

BERG, J. M. and KIRMAN, B. H. 1961. "Risk of dual occurrence of mongolism in sibships." *Arch. Dis. Child.* 36: 645–48.

BERG, J. M. and STERN, J. 1963. "Observations on children with mongolism." *Proc. Second International Congress on Mental Retardation, Part I,* pp. 367–72.

BERNHARD, W. G., GORE, I., and KILBY, R. A. 1951. "Congenital leukemia." *Blood* 6: 990–1001.

Bixby, E. M. 1939. "Biochemical studies in mongolism." *Amer. J. Ment. Defic.* 44: 59.

———. 1940. "Further biochemical studies in mongolism." *Amer. J. Ment. Defic.* 45: 201–06.

Bixby, E. M. and Benda, C. E. 1942–43. "Glucose tolerance and insulin tolerance in mongolism." *Amer. J. Ment. Defic.* 47: 158–66.

Blaha, G. C. 1964. "Effect of age of the donor and recipient on the development of transferred golden hamster ova." *Anat. Rec.* 150: 413–16.

Blandau, R. J. 1952. "The female factor in fertility and infertility. I. Effects of delayed fertilization on the development of the pronuclei in rat ova." *Fertil. & Steril.* 3: 349–62.

Bleyer, A. 1934. "Indications that mongoloid imbecility is a gametic mutation of degressive type." *Amer. J. Dis. Child.* 47: 342–48.

Blumberg, B. S., Gerstley, B. J. S., Hungerford, D. A., London, W. T., and Sutnick, A. I. 1967. "A serum antigen (Australia antigen) in Down's syndrome, leukemia, and hepatitis." *Ann. Int. Med.* 66: 924–31.

Bodian, M. and Carter, C. O. 1963. "A family study of Hirschsprung's disease." *Ann. Hum. Genet.* 26: 261–77.

Böök, J. A. and Reed, S. C. 1950. "Empiric risk figures in mongolism." *J.A.M.A.* 143: 730–32.

Brandt, N. 1962. "Genes on the mongol chromosome?" *Lancet* 2: 837.

Brandt, N. J., Frøland, A., Mikkelsen, M., Nielsen, A., and Tolstrup, N. 1963. "Galactosaemia locus and the Down's syndrome chromosome." *Lancet* 2: 700–03.

Breg, W. R., Miller, O. J., and Schmickel, R. D. 1962. "Chromosomal translocations in patients with mongolism and in their normal relatives." *New Eng. J. Med.* 266: 845–52.

Brewis, M., Poskanzer, D. C., Rolland, C., and Miller, H. 1966. "Neurological disease in an English city." *Acta Neurol. Scand. Suppl. 24,* 42: 1–89.

Brewster, H. F. and Cannon, H. E. 1930. "Acute lymphatic leukemia: Report of case in eleventh month mongolian idiot." *New Orleans Med. Surg. J.* 82: 872–73.

Bridges, C. B. 1916. "Non-disjunction as proof of the chromosome theory of heredity." *Genetics* 1: 1–52, 107–63.

Brochier, A. 1947. "Fréquence du mongolisme chez le nouveau-né: Pronostic vital chez les enfants mongoliens du premier âge." *Pediatrie* 2: 437–38.

Brøgger, A., Mohr, J., Wehn, M., and Vislie, H. 1964. "Concerning translocation as a cause of mental retardation," in: *Proc. International Copenhagen Congress on the Scientific Study of Mental Retardation,* vol. I, pp. 128–31.

Brousseau, K. and Brainerd, H. G. 1928. *Mongolism: A Study of the Physical and Mental Characteristics of Mongolian Imbeciles.* London: Bailliere, Tindall, and Cox.

Buchan, A. R. 1962. "A study of mongolism in Newcastle-upon-Tyne 1948–1959." *Med. Off.* 107: 51–54.

Buck, C., Valentine, G. H., and Hamilton, K. "Reproductive performance of mothers of mongols." *Amer. J. Ment. Defic.* 70: 886–94.

Buckton, K. E., Harnden, D. G., Baikie, A. G., and Woods, G. E. 1961. "Mongolism and leukaemia in the same sibship." *Lancet* 1: 171–72.

Burgio, G. R., Severi, F., Rossoni, R., and Vaccaro, R. 1966. "Autoantibodies in Down's syndrome." *Lancet* 1: 497–98.

Butcher, R. L. and Fugo, N. W. 1967. "Overripeness and the mammalian ova, II. Delayed ovulation and chromosome anomalies." *Fertil. & Steril.* 18: 297–302.

Cannings, C. and Cannings, M. R. 1968. "Mongolism, delayed fertilization and human sexual behavior." *Nature* 218: 481.

Cantolino, S. J., Schmickel, R. D., Bail, M., and Cisar, C. F. 1966. "Persistent chromosomal aberrations following radioiodine therapy for thyrotoxicosis." *New Eng. J. Med.* 275: 739–45.

Carr, D. H. 1963. "Chromosome studies in abortuses and stillborn infants." *Lancet* 2: 603–06.

———. 1967. "Chromosome anomalies as a cause of spontaneous abortion." *Amer. J. Obstet. Gynec.* 97: 283–93.

Carter, C. and MacCarthy, D. 1951. "Incidence of mongolism and its diagnosis in the newborn." *Brit. J. Soc. Med.* 5: 83–90.

Carter, C. O. 1958. "A life-table for mongols with the causes of death." *J. Ment. Defic.* 2: 64–74.

Carter, C. O. and Evans, K. A. 1961 "Risk of parents who have had one child with Down's syndrome (mongolism) having another child similarly affected." *Lancet* 2: 785–88.

Carter, C. O., Evans, K. A., and Stewart, A. M. 1961. "Maternal radiation and Down's syndrome (mongolism)." *Lancet* 2: 1042.

Carter, C. O., Hamerton, J. L., Polani, P. E., Gunalp, A., and Weller, S. D. V. 1960. "Chromosome translocation as a cause of familial mongolism." *Lancet* 2: 678–80.

Ceccarelli, G. and Torbidoni, L. 1967. "Viral hepatitis and Down's syndrome." *Lancet* 1: 438.

Chapman, M. J. and Stern, J. Cited in: Penrose, L. S. and Smith, G. F. 1966. *Down's Anomaly.* Boston: Little, Brown and Company.

Chitham, R. G. and MacIver, E. 1965. "A cytogenetic and statistical survey of 105 cases of mongolism." *Ann. Hum. Genet.* 28: 309–15.

Clendenin, T. M. and Benirschke, K. 1963. "Chromosome studies on spontaneous abortions." *Lab. Invest.* 12: 1281–92.

Collmann, R. D. and Stoller, A. 1962. "A survey of mongoloid births in Victoria, Australia, 1942–1957." *Amer. J. Public Health* 52: 813–29.

———. 1963*a*. "Comparison of age distributions for mothers of mongols born in high and in low birth incidence areas and years in Victoria, 1942–57." *J. Ment. Defic. Res.* 7: 79–83.

———. 1963*b*. "A life-table for mongols in Victoria, Australia." *J. Ment. Defic. Res.* 7: 53–59.

CONEN, P. E., ERKMAN, B., and LASKI, B. 1966. "Chromosome studies on a radiographer and her family." *Arch Intern. Med.* 117: 125–32.

COPPEN, A. and COWIE, V. 1960. "Maternal health and mongolism." *Brit. Med. J.* 1: 1843–47.

COWIE, V. 1961. "Maternal constitution and mongolism." *Proc. Second International Congress on Human Genetics* 2: 1080–82.

COWIE, V. A. 1966. "Chromosomal findings in a population-based sample of mongols." *Ala. J. Med. Sci.* 3: 493–95.

COWIE, V. and SLATER, E. 1963. "Maternal age and miscarriage in the mothers of mongols." *Acta Genet.* 13: 77–83.

DALLAIRE, L. and KINGS-MILL FLYNN, D. 1967*a*. "Infectious hepatitis and Down's syndrome." *Lancet* 2: 467.

DALLAIRE, L. and FLYNN, D. 1967b. "Frequency of antibodies to thyroglobulin in relation to gravidity and to Down's syndrome." *Canad. Med. Assoc. J.* 97: 209–12.

DAVIDENKOVA, E. F., SHTIL'BANS, I. I., GODINOVA, A. M., SAVEL'EVA-VASIL'EVA, E. A., and BERLINSKAYA, D. K. 1964. "Role of maternal pathology in Down's disease." *Fed. Proc. Trans. Suppl.* 23: 873–75.

DAVIES, A. M. 1968. Personal communication.

DAY, R. W. 1966. "The epidemiology of chromosome aberrations." *Amer. J. Hum. Genet.* 18: 70–80.

DAY, R. W. and WRIGHT, S. W. 1965. "Down's syndrome at young maternal ages: Chromosomal and family studies." *J. Pediat.* 66: 764–71.

DEKABAN, A. 1965. "Twins, probably monozygotic: One mongoloid with 48 chromosomes, the other normal." *Cytogenetics* 4: 227–39.

DEKABAN, A. S., BENDER, M. A., and ECONOMOS, G. E. 1963. "Chromosome studies in mongoloids and their families." *Cytogenetics* 2: 61–75.

DEWOLFF, E. 1964. "Etude clinique de 134 mongoliens." *Ann. Paed. Suppl.* 202: 1–47.

DEWOLFF, E., SCHÄRER, K., and LEJEUNE, J. 1962. "Contribution à l'étude des juneaux mongoliens: Un cas de monozygotisme hétérocaryote." *Helv. Paed.* 17: 301–28.

DONNELL, G. N., NG, W. G., BERGREN, W. R., MELNYK, J., and KOCH, R. 1965. "Enhancement of erythrocyte-galactokinase activity in Langdon-Down trisomy." *Lancet* 1: 553.

DONNER, M. 1954. "A study of the immunology and biology of mongolism." *Ann. Med. Exp. Biol. Fenn.*, Suppl. 9, 32: 1–80.

DOWN, J. LANGDON, H. 1867. "Observations on ethnic classification of idiots." *J. Ment. Sci.* 13: 121–23.

DRILLIEN, C. M. and WILKINSON, E. M. 1964. "Emotional stress and mongoloid births." *Develop. Med. Child Neurol.* 6: 140–43.

DUTTON, G. 1959. "The neutrol 17-ketosteroid and 17-ketogenic steroid excretion of mongol and non-mongol mentally defective boys." *J. Ment. Defic. Res.* 3: 103–07.

EDGREN, J., DE LA CHAPELLE, A., and KÄÄRIÄINEN, R. 1966. "Cytogenetic study of seventy-three patients with Down's syndrome." *J. Ment. Defic. Res.* 10: 47–62.

EDWARDS, J. H., DENT, T., and GULI, E. 1963. "Sporadic mongols with translocations." *Lancet* 2: 902.

EK, J. I. 1959. "Thyroid function in mothers of mongoloid infants." *Acta Paed.* 48: 33–42.

EK, J. I. and JENSEN, M. K. 1959. Cited in: COWIE, V., 1961. "Maternal constitution and mongolism." *Proc. Second International Congress on Human Genetics* 2: 1080–82.

EMANUEL, B., PADORR, M. P., and SWENSON, O. 1965. "Mongolism associated with Hirschsprung's disease." *J. Pediat.* 66: 437–39.

ENGEL, E. 1967. "Auto-antibodies and chromosomal aberrations." *Lancet* 1: 1271–72.

ENGEL, R. R., HAMMOND, D., EITZMAN, D. V., PEARSON, H., and KRIVIT, W. 1964. "Transient congenital leukemia in 7 infants with mongolism." *J. Pediat.* 65: 303–05.

FIALKOW, P. J. 1966. "Autoimmunity and chromosomal aberrations." *Amer. J. Hum. Genet.* 18: 93–108.

———. 1967. "Thyroid antibodies, Down's syndrome, and maternal age." *Nature* 214: 1253–54.

FIALKOW, P. J., UCHIDA, I. A., HECHT, F., and MOTULSKY, A. G. 1965. "Increased frequency of thyroid autoantibodies in mothers of patients with Down's syndrome." *Lancet* 2: 868–70.

FLUCK, E. R. 1962. "Biochemical studies in mongolism: Structures of gamma-globulins from mongoloid blood." Thesis, Ph.D., Pennsylvania State University.

FORD, C. E. 1962. "Human chromosomes," in: *Chromosomes in Medicine.* Little Club Clinics in Developmental Medicine No. 5, pp. 47–58. London: Spastics Soc. Heinemann.

FORD, C. E., JONES, K. W., MILLER, O. J., MITTWOCH, U., PENROSE, L. S., RIDLER, M., and SHAPIRO, A. 1959. "The chromosomes in a patient showing both mongolism and the Klinefelter syndrome." *Lancet* 1: 709–10.

FORSSMAN, H. and ÅKESSON, H. O. 1965. "Mortality in patients with Down's syndrome." *J. Ment. Defic. Res.* 9: 146–49.

———. 1967. "Consanguineous marriages and mongolism," in: Ciba Foundation Study Group No. 25, *Mongolism,* pp. 23–34. Boston: Little, Brown and Company.

FORSSMAN, H. and LEHMANN, O. 1962. "Chromosome studies in eleven families with mongolism in more than one member." *Acta Paed.* 51: 180–88.

FRAUMENI, J. F., JR., and MILLER, R. W. 1967. "Epidemiology of human leukemia: Recent observations." *J. Nat. Cancer Inst.* 38: 593–605.

FUGO, N. W. and BUTCHER, R. L. 1966. "Overripeness and the mammalian ova." *Fertil. & Steril.* 17: 804–14.

FULLER, R. W., LUCE, M. W., and MERTZ, E. T. 1962. "Serum uric acid in mongolism." *Science* 137: 868–69.

GENTRY, J. T., PARKHURST, E., and BULIN, G. V., JR. 1959. "An epidemiological study of congenital malformations in New York State." *Amer. J. Public Health* 49: 497–513.

GERMAN, J. 1968. "Mongolism, delayed fertilization, and human sexual behavior." *Nature* 217: 516–18.

GERSHOFF, S. N., HEGSTED, D. M., and TRULSON, M. F. 1958. "Metabolic studies of mongoloids." *Amer. J. Clin. Nutr.* 6: 526–30.

GOODMAN, H. O., LOFLAND, H. B., and THOMAS, J. J. 1966–67. "Serum uric acid levels in mongolism." *Amer. J. Ment. Defic.* 71: 437–46.

GORDON, H., TORRINGTON, M., LOUW, J. H., and CYWES, S. 1966. "A genetical study of Hirschsprung's disease: Congenital intestinal aganglionosis." *S. Afr. Med. J.* 40: 720–21.

GRAIVIER, L. and SIEBER, W. K. 1966. "Hirschsprung's disease and mongolism." *Surgery* 60: 458–61.

GREENBERG, R. C. 1963. "Two factors influencing the births of mongols to younger mothers." *Med. Off.* 109: 62–64.

GUSTAVSON, K. H. 1964. *Down's Syndrome: A Clinical and Cytogenetical Investigation.* Uppsala: Almqvist and Wiksell.

HACKEL, E. 1954. "Blood factor incompatibility in the etiology of mental deficiency." *Amer. J. Hum. Genet.* 6: 224–40.

HALEVI, H. S. 1967. "Congenital malformations in Israel." *Brit. J. Prev. Soc. Med.* 21: 66–77.

HALL, B. 1964. "Mongolism in newborns: A clinical and cytogenetic study." *Acta Paed. Suppl.* 154: 1–95.

HALL, B. and KALLEN, B. 1964. "Chromosome studies in abortuses and stillborn infants." *Lancet* 1: 110–11.

HAMERTON, J. L. 1962. "Cytogenetics of mongolism," in: *Chromosomes in Medicine.* Little Club Clinics in Developmental Medicine No. 5, pp. 140–82. London: Spastics Soc. Heinemann.

HAMERTON, J. L., BRIGGS, S. M., GIANNELLI, F., and CARTER, C. O. 1961. "Chromosome studies in detection of parents with high risk of second child with Down's syndrome." *Lancet* 2: 788–91.

HAMERTON, J. L., GIANNELLI, F., and POLANI, P. E. 1965. "Cytogenetics of Down's syndrome (mongolism) I. Data on a consecutive series of patients referred for genetic counselling and diagnosis." *Cytogenetics* 4: 171–85.

HAMERTON, J. L., JAGIELLO, G. M., and KIRMAN, B. H. 1962. "Sex-chromosome abnormalities in a population of mentally defective children." *Brit. Med. J.* 1: 220–23.

HAMERTON, J. L., TAYLOR, A. I., ANGELL, R., and MCGUIRE, V. M. 1965. "Chromosome investigations of a small isolated human population: Chromosome abnormalities and distribution of chromosome counts according to age and sex among the population of Tristan da Cunha." *Nature* 206: 1232–34.

HARNDEN, D. G. 1962. "Normal and abnormal cell division," in: *Chromosomes in Medicine.* Little Club Clinics in Developmental Medicine No. 5, pp. 17–34. London: Spastics Soc. Heinemann.

HARNDEN, D. G., MILLER, O. J., and PENROSE, L. S. 1960. "The Klinefelter-mongolism type of double aneuploidy." *Ann. Hum. Genet.* 24: 165–68.

HARRIS, L. E. and STEINBERG, A. G. 1954. "Abnormalities observed during the first six days of life in 8,716 live-born infants." *Pediatrics* 14: 314–26.

HASHEM, N. and SAKR, R. 1963. "Mongolism among Egyptian children." *Proc. Second International Congress on Mental Retardation, 1961, Part I,* pp. 387–403.

HAYASHI, T. 1962. Cited in: STARKMAN, M. N. and SHAW, M. W. 1967. "Atypical acrocentric chromosomes in Negro and Caucasian mongols." *Amer. J. Hum. Genet.* 19: 162–73.

———. 1963. "Karyotypic analysis of 83 cases of Down's syndrome in Harris County, Texas." *Tex. Rep. Biol. Med.* 21: 28–36.

HAYLES, A. B., HINRICHS, W. L., and TAUXE, W. N. 1965. "Thyroid disease among children with Down's syndrome (mongolism)." *Pediatrics* 36: 608–14.

HAYS, D. M. and NORRIS, W. J. 1956. "Congenital aganglionic megacolon." *Calif. Med.* 84: 403–06.

HEATH, C. W., JR., and MOLONEY, W. C. 1965. "Familial leukemia: Five cases of acute leukemia in three generations." *New Eng. J. Med.* 272: 882–87.

HECHT, F., BRYANT, J. S., MOTULSKY, A. G., and GIBLETT, E. R. 1963. "The no. 17–18 (E) trisomy syndrome: Studies on cytogenetics dermatoglyphics, paternal age, and linkage." *J. Pediat.* 63: 605–21.

HEDBERG, E., HOLMDAHL, K., PEHRSON, S., and ZACKRISSON, U. 1963. "On relationship between maternal conditions during pregnancy and congenital malformations." *Acta Paed.* 52: 353–60.

HEINRICHS, E. H., ALLEN, S. W., JR., NELSON, P. S. 1963. "Simultaneous 18-trisomy and 21-trisomy cluster." *Lancet* 2: 468.

HOFMANN, S. and REHBEIN, F. 1966. "Hirschsprungsche krankheit im neugeborenenalter." *Ztschr. f. Kinderchir.* 3: 182–94.

HOLLAND, W. W., DOLL, R., and CARTER, C. O. 1962. "The mortality from leukaemia and other cancers among patients with Down's syndrome (mongols) and among their parents." *Brit. J. Cancer* 16: 177–86.

HSIA, D. Y.-Y., INOUYE, T., WONG, P., and SOUTH, A. 1964. "Studies on galactose oxidation in Down's syndrome." *New Eng. J. Med.* 270: 1085–88.

HUANG, S. W., EMANUEL, I., LO, J., LIAO, S.-K., and HSU, C.-C. 1967. "A cytogenetic study of 77 Chinese children with Down's syndrome." *J. Ment. Defic. Res.* 11: 147–52.

HUG, V. E. 1951. "Das geschlechtsverhältnis beim mongolismus." *Ann. Paed.* 177: 31–54.

HUSTINX, T. W. J., EBERLE, P., GEERTS, S. J., BRINK, J. T., and WOLTRING, L. M. 1961. "Mongoloid twins with 48 chromosomes (AA + A_{21}, XXY)." *Ann. Hum. Genet.* 25: 111–15.

HUTTON, A. C. and SMITH, G. F. 1964. "Haptoglobins and transferrins in patients with Down's syndrome." *Ann. Hum. Genet.* 27: 413–15.

INGALLS, T. H. 1947*a*. "Etiology of mongolism: Epidemiologic and teratologic implications." *Amer. J. Dis. Child.* 74: 147–65.

———. 1947*b*. "Pathogenesis of mongolism." *Amer. J. Dis. Child.* 73: 279–92.

INGALLS, T. H., BABBOTT, J., and PHILBROOK, R. 1957. "The mothers of mongoloid babies: A retrospective appraisal of their health during pregnancy." *Amer. J. Obstet. Gynec.* 74: 572–81.

INGALLS, T. H. and GORDON, J. E. 1947. "Epidemiologic implications of developmental arrests." *Amer. J. Med. Sci.* 214: 322–28.

INGALLS, T. H. and HENRY, T. A. 1968. "Trisomy and D/G translocation mongolism in brothers." *New Eng. J. Med.* 278: 10–14.

IVERSON, T. 1966. "Leukaemia in infancy and childhood—a material of 570 Danish cases." *Acta Paed. Scand. Suppl.* 167–70.

JACOBS, P. A., BRUNTON, M., COURT-BROWN, W. M., DOLL, R., and GOLDSTEIN, H. 1963. "Change of human chromosome count distributions with age: Evidence for a sex difference." *Nature* 197: 1080–81.

JAGIELLO, G., KARNICKI, J., and RYAN, R. J. 1968. "Superovulation with pituitary gonadotrophins: Method for obtaining meiotic metaphase figures in human ova." *Lancet* 1: 178–80.

JAGIELLO, G. and TAYLOR, M. B. 1965. "Chromosomal studies of two cases of trisomy-21 Down's syndrome with hyperthyroidism." *Amer. J. Ment. Defic.* 69: 645–48.

JENKINS, R. L. 1933. "Etiology of mongolism." *Amer. J. Dis. Child.* 45: 506–19.

JÉRÔME, H. 1962. "Anomalies du métabolisme du tryptophane dans la maladie mongolienne." *Bull. Mem. Soc. Med. Hop. Paris* 113: 168–72.

JÉRÔME, H., LEJEUNE, J., and TURPIN, R. 1960. "Étude de l'excrétion urinaire de certains métabolites du tryptophane chez les enfants mongoliens." *C. R. Acad. Sci.* 251: 474–76.

JOHNSTON, A. W. and JASLOW, R. I. 1963. "Children of mothers with Down's syndrome." *New Eng. J. Med.* 269: 439–43.

KAHN, E. Cited in: LUDER, J. and MUSOKE, L. K. 1955. "Mongolism in Africans." *Arch. Dis. Child.* 30: 310–15.

KARHAUSEN, L. W. and HUTCHISON, G. B. Cited in: MILLER, R. W. 1966. "Relation between cancer and congenital defects in man." *New Eng. J. Med.* 275: 87–93.

KAY, C. J. and ESSELBORN, V. M. 1963. "Hyperthyroidism and mongolism." *Amer. J. Dis. Child.* 106: 121–24.

KING, J. S., JR., GOODMAN, H. O., and THOMAS, J. J. 1966. "Urinary amino acid excretion in mongolism." *Acta Genet.* (Basel) 16: 132–54.

KING, M. J., GILLIS, E. M., and BAIKIE, A. G. 1962. "The polymorph alkaline phosphatase in mongolism." *Lancet* 2: 661.

KNOX, G. 1963. "Detection of low intensity epidemicity application to cleft lip and palate." *Brit. J. Prev. Soc. Med.* 17: 121–27.

———. 1964. "Epidemiology of childhood leukaemia in Northumberland and Durham." *Brit. J. Prev. Soc. Med.* 18: 17–24.

KOGON, A., KRONMAL, R., and PETERSON, D. R. 1967. "Viral hepatitis and Down's syndrome." *Lancet* 1: 615.

———. 1968. "The relationship between infectious hepatitis and Down's syndrome." *Amer. J. Public Health,* 58: 305–11.

KRIVIT, W. and GOOD, R. A. 1957. "Simultaneous occurrence of mongolism and leukemia: Report of a nationwide survey." *A.M.A. J. Dis. Child.* 94: 289–93.

KRONE, W., WOLF, U., GOEDDE, H. W., and BAITSCH, H. 1964. "Enhancement of erythrocyte-galactokinase activity in Langdon-Down trisomy." *Lancet* 2: 590.

KURLAND, L. T. 1958. "Descriptive epidemiology of selected neurologic and myopathic disorders with particular reference to a survey in Rochester, Minnesota." *J. Chronic Dis.* 8: 378–418.

KWITEROVICH, P. O., JR., CROSS, H. E., and MCKUSICK, V. A. 1966. "Mongolism in an inbred population." *Bull. Johns Hopkins Hosp.* 119: 268–75.

LANDER, E., FORSSMAN, H., and ÅKESSON, H. O. 1964. "Season of birth and mental deficiency." *Acta Genet.* (Basel) 14: 265–80.

LANDTMAN, B. 1948. "On the relationship between maternal conditions during pregnancy and congenital malformations." *Arch. Dis. Child.* 23: 237–46.

LANG-BROWN, H., LAWLER, S. D., and PENROSE, L. S. 1952–53. "The blood typing of cases of mongolism, their parents and sibs." *Ann. Eugen.* 17: 307–36.

LANMAN, J. T., SKLARIN, B. S., COOPER, H. L., and HIRSCHHORN, K. 1960. "Klinefelter's syndrome in a ten-month-old mongolian idiot." *New Eng. J. Med.* 263: 887–90.

LECK, I. 1966. "Incidence and epidemicity of Down's syndrome." *Lancet* 2: 457–60.

LEHMANN, O. and FORSSMAN, H. 1960. "Klinefelter's syndrome and mongolism in the same person." *Acta Paed.* 49: 536–39.

LEJEUNE, J. 1964. "The 21 trisomy—Current stage of chromosomal research." *Progr. Med. Genet.* 3: 144–72.

LEJEUNE, J., GAUTIER, M., and TURPIN, R. 1959*a*. "Étude des chromosomes somatiques de neuf enfants mongoliens." *C. R. Acad. Sci.* 248: 1721–22.

———. 1959*b*. "Les chromosomes humains en culture de tissus." *C. R. Acad. Sci.* 248: 602–03.

LENNOX, B., WHITE, H. ST. C., and CAMPBELL, J. 1962. "The polymorph alkaline phosphatase in mongolism." *Lancet* 2: 991–92.

LEVINSON, A., FRIEDMAN, A., and STAMPS, F. 1955. "Variability of mongolism." *Pediatrics* 16: 43–54.

LILIENFELD, A. M. 1966. "Epidemiological studies of the leukemogenic effects of radiation." *Yale J. Biol. Med.* 39: 143–64.

LILIENFELD, A. M., PEDERSON, E., and DOWD, J. E. 1967. *Cancer Epidemiology: Methods of Study*. Baltimore: The Johns Hopkins Press.

LÜERS, T. and LÜERS, H. 1954. "Über eine segmentierungshemmung der neutrophilen leukocyten bei mongolismus." *Artz. Forsch.* 8: 263–67.

LUNDIN, L. G. and GUSTAVSON, K. H. 1962. "Urinary BAIB excretion in Down's syndrome (mongolism)." *Acta Genet.* 12: 156–63.

LUNN, J. E. 1959. "A survey of mongol children in Glasgow." *Scot. Med. J.* 4: 368–72.

MAAS, J. W. 1964. "Some biochemical data on children with mongolism," in: *Proc. International Copenhagen Congress on the Scientific Study of Mental Retardation,* vol. 1, pp. 211–14.

MACLEAN, N., MITCHELL, J. M., HARNDEN, D. G., WILLIAMS, J., JACOBS, P. A., BUCKTON, K. A., BAIKIE, A. G., COURT-BROWN, W. M., MCBRIDE, J. A., STRONG, J. A., CLOSE, H. G., and JONES, D. C. 1962. "A survey of sex-chromosome abnormalities among 4,514 mental defectives." *Lancet* 1: 293–96.

MACMAHON, B., PUGH, T. F., and IPSEN, J. 1960. *Epidemiologic Methods.* Boston: Little, Brown and Company.

MADSEN, C. M. 1964. *Hirschsprung's Disease.* Copenhagen: Munksgaard.

MAKINO, S. 1964. "Chromosomal studies in normal human subjects and in 300 cases of congenital disorders." Parts I, II, and III. *Cytologia* 29: 12–262.

MAKINO, S., KIKUCHI, Y., SASAKI, M. S., SASAKI, M., and YOSHIDA, M. 1962. "A further survey of the chromosomes in the Japanese." *Chromosoma* 13: 148–62.

MALPAS, P. 1937. "The incidence of human malformations and the significance of changes in the maternal environment in their causation." *J. Obstet. Gynec.* 44: 434–54.

MANTEL, N. 1967. "The detection of disease clustering and a generalized regression approach." *Cancer Res.* 27: 209–20.

MANTEL, N. and STARK, C. R. 1966–67. "Paternal age in Down's syndrome." *Amer. J. Ment. Defic.* 71: 1025.

MATSUNAGA, E. 1963. "Down's syndrome in Japan." *Nat. Inst. Genet. Ann. Rep.* 14: 128–30.

———. 1966. "Down's syndrome and maternal inbreeding." *Acta Genet. Med. Gemell.* 15: 224–30.

———. 1967*a*. General discussion in: Ciba Foundation Study Group No. 25, *Mongolism,* pp. 88–95. Boston: Little, Brown and Company.

———. 1967*b*. "Parental age, live-birth order and pregnancy-free interval in Down's syndrome in Japan," in: Ciba Foundation Study Group No. 25, *Mongolism,* pp. 6–22. Boston: Little, Brown and Company.

MAVOR, J. W. 1924. "The production of non-disjunction by X-rays." *J. Exp. Zool.* 39: 381–432.

MCCOY, E. E. and CHUNG, S. I. 1964. "The excretion of tryptophan metabolites following deoxypyriodoxine administration in mongoloid and nonmongoloid patients." *J. Pediat.* 64: 227–33.

MCDONALD, A. D. 1961. "Maternal health in early pregnancy and congenital defect: Final report on a prospective inquiry." *Brit. J. Prev. Soc. Med.* 15: 154–66.

McIntosh, R., Merritt, K. K., Richards, M. R., Samuels, M. H., and Bellows, M. T. 1954. "The incidence of congenital malformations: A study of 5,964 pregnancies." *Pediatrics* 14: 505–21.

Mella, B. and Lang, D. J. 1967. "Leukocyte mitosis: Suppression in vitro associated with acute infectious hepatitis." *Science* 155: 80–81.

Mellman, W. J., Oski, F. A., Tedesco, T. A., Maciera-Coelho, A., and Harris, H. 1964. "Leucocyte enzymes in Down's syndrome." *Lancet* 2: 674.

Mellon, J. P., Pay, B. Y., and Green, D. M. 1963. "Mongolism and thyroid auto-antibodies." *J. Ment. Defic. Res.* 7: 31–37.

Mercer, R. D., Keller, M. K., and Lansdale, D. 1963. "An extra abnormal chromosome in a child with mongolism and acute myeloblastic leukemia." *Cleveland Clin. Quart.* 30: 215–24.

Merrit, D. H. and Harris, J. S. 1956. "Mongolism and acute leukemia: A report of four cases." *A.M.A. J. Dis. Child.* 92: 41–44.

Mertz, E. T., Fuller, R. W., and Concon, J. M. 1963. "Serum uric acid in young mongoloids." *Science* 141: 535.

Migeon, B. R. 1965. Cited in: Starkman, M. N. and Shaw, M. W. 1967. "Atypical acrocentric chromosomes in Negro and Caucasian mongols." *Amer. J. Hum. Genet.* 19: 162–73.

Migeon, B. R., Kaufmann, B. N., and Young, W. J. 1962. "A chromosome abnormality with fragment in a paramongol child." *Bull. Johns Hopkins Hosp.* 111: 221–29.

Mikkelsen, M. and Frøland, A. 1964. "Sex chromatin in patients with Down's syndrome (mongolism)," in: *Proc. International Copenhagen Congress on the Scientific Study of Mental Retardation (2nd Conf.),* pp. 162–64.

Milham, S., Jr., and Gittelsohn, A. M. 1965. "Parental age and malformations." *Hum. Biol.* 37: 13–22.

Miller, J. R. and Dill, F. J. 1965. "The cytogenetics of mongolism," in: *International Psychiatry Clinics,* vol. 2, no. 1, pp. 127–52.

Miller, O. J., Breg, W. R., Schmickel, R. D., and Tretter, W. 1961. "A family with an XXXXY male, a leukaemic male, and two 21-trisomic mongoloid females." *Lancet* 2: 78–79.

Miller, R. W. 1963. "Down's syndrome (mongolism), other congenital malformations and cancers among the sibs of leukemic children." *New Eng. J. Med.* 268: 393–401.

———. 1966. "Relation between cancer and congenital defects in man." *New Eng. J. Med.* 275: 87–93.

Mittwoch, U. 1957. "Some observations on the leucocytes in mongolism." *J. Ment. Defic. Res.* 1: 26–31.

Nelson, T. L. 1961. "Serum protein and lipoprotein fractions in mongolism." *Amer. J. Dis. Child.* 102: 369–74.

Nichols, W. W. 1966. "The role of viruses in the etiology of chromosomal abnormalities." *Amer. J. Hum. Genet.* 18: 81–92.

O'BRIEN, D. and GROSHEK, A. 1962. "The abnormality of tryptophane metabolism in children with mongolism." *Arch. Dis. Child.* 37: 17–20.

O'BRIEN, D., ZARINS, B., and JENSEN, C. B. 1962. "The abnormality of tryptophan metabolism in children with mongolism: Studies following 3-hydroxy-DL-kynuerenine administration." *Proc. Cong. Amer. Soc. Pediat. Res.,* p. 122.

O'LEARY, W. D. 1931. "Carbohydrate metabolism in mongolian idiots as evidence of endocrine dysfunction." *Amer. J. Dis. Child.* 41: 544–51.

ØSTER, J. 1953. *Mongolism. A Clinicogenealogical Investigation Comprising 526 Mongols Living on Seeland and Neighbouring Islands in Denmark.* Copenhagen: Danish Science Press.

_______. 1956. "The causes of mongolism." *Dan. Med. Bull.* 3: 158–64.

ØSTER, J., MIKKELSEN, M., and NIELSEN, A. 1964. "The mortality and causes of death in patients with Down's syndrome (mongolism)," in: *Proc. International Copenhagen Congress on the Scientific Study of Mental Retardation,* vol. 1, pp. 231–35.

O'SULLIVAN, J. B., REDDY, W. J., and FARRELL, M. J. 1961. "Adrenal function in mongolism." *Amer. J. Dis. Child.* 101: 37–40.

PARKER, G. F. 1950. "The incidence of mongoloid imbecility in the newborn infant: A ten-year study covering 27,931 live births." *J. Pediat.* 36: 493–94.

PASSARGE, E. 1967. "The genetics of Hirschsprung's disease: Evidence for heterogeneous etiology and a study of sixty-three families." *New Eng. J. Med.* 276: 138–43.

PENROSE, L. S. 1932. "The blood grouping of mongolian imbeciles." *Lancet* 1: 394–95.

_______. 1934. "The relative aetiological importance of birth order and maternal age in mongolism." *Proc. Roy. Soc. Lond.* 115: 431–50.

_______. 1934–35. "A method of separating the relative aetiological effects of birth order and maternal age, with special reference to mongolian imbecility." *Ann. Eugen.* 6: 108–22.

_______. 1939. "Maternal age, order of birth and developmental abnormalities." *J. Ment. Sci.* 85: 1141–50.

_______. 1949. "The incidence of mongolism in the general population." *J. Ment. Sci.* 95: 685.

_______. 1962. "Paternal age in mongolism." *Lancet* 1: 1101.

_______. 1965. "The causes of Down's syndrome," in: *Advances in Teratology.* London: Logos Press.

PENROSE, L. S. and BERG, J. M. 1968. "Mongolism and duration of marriage." *Nature* 218: 300.

PENROSE, L. S., ELLIS, J. R., and DELHANTY, J. D. A. 1960. "Chromosomal translocations in mongolism and in normal relatives." *Lancet* 2: 409–10.

PENROSE, L. S. and SMITH, G. F. 1966. *Down's Anomaly.* Boston: Little, Brown and Company.

PERRY, T. L., SHAW, K. N. F., and WALKER, D. 1959. "Urinary excretion of B-amino-isobutyric acid in mongolism." *Nature* 184: 1970.

PETERSEN, C. D. and LUZZATTI, L. 1965. "The role of chromosome translocation in the recurrence risk of Down's syndrome." *Pediatrics* 35: 463–69.

PLEYDELL, M. J. 1957. "Mongolism and other congenital abnormalities: An epidemiological study in Northamptonshire." *Lancet* 1: 1314–19.

POLANI, P. E. Discussion in: FORSSMAN, H. and ÅKESSON, H. O. 1967. "Consanguineous marriages and mongolism." Ciba Foundation Study Group No. 25, *Mongolism,* pp. 23–34. Boston: Little, Brown and Company.

POLANI, P. E., FORD, C. E., BRIGGS, J. H., and CLARKE, C. M. 1960. "A mongol girl with 46 chromosomes." *Lancet* 1: 721–24.

POZSONYI, J. and GIBSON, D. 1965–66. "Biochemical consequences of supernumerary chromosome subtype in mongolism." *Amer. J. Ment. Defic.* 70: 213–17.

PRITHAM, G. H., APPLETON, M. D., and FLUCK, E. R. 1962–63. "Biochemical studies in mongolism, I. The influence of environment on the concentrations and mobilities of plasma proteins." *Amer. J. Ment. Defic.* 67: 517–20.

RAPAPORT, I. 1963. "Mongolian oligophrenia and dental caries." *Rev. Stomat.* 64: 207–18.

RECORD, R. G. and SMITH, A. 1955. "Incidence, mortality, and sex distribution of mongoloid defectives." *Brit. J. Prev. Soc. Med.* 9: 10–15.

REISS, M., WAKOH, T., HILLMAN, J. C., PEARSE, J. J., DALEY, N., and REISS, J. M. 1965–66. "Endocrine investigations into mongolism." *Amer. J. Ment. Defic.* 70: 204–12.

RENWICK, D. H. G., MILLER, J. R., and PATERSON, D. 1964. "Estimates of incidence and prevalence of mongolism and of congenital heart disease in British Columbia." *Canad. Med. Assoc. J.* 91: 365–71.

RICHARDS, B. W., STEWART, A., SYLVESTER, P. E., and JASIEWICZ, V. 1965. "Cytogenetic survey of 225 patients diagnosed clinically as mongols." *J. Ment. Defic. Res.* 9: 245–59.

ROBINSON, A. and PUCK, T. T. 1967. "Studies on chromosomal nondisjunction in man. II." *Amer. J. Hum. Genet.* 19: 112–29.

ROBSON, H. N. 1962. "Human chromosomal abnormalities." *Aust. Ann. Med.* 11: 281–90.

ROHDE, R. A. 1965. "Congenital chromosomal syndromes: A model for pathogenesis." *Calif. Med.* 103: 249–53.

ROSNER, F., ONG, B. H., PAINE, R. S., and MAHANAND, D. 1965*a*. "Biochemical differentiation of trisomic Down's syndrome (mongolism) from that due to translocation." *New Eng. J. Med.* 273: 1356–61.

———. 1965*b*. "Blood-serotonin activity in trisomic and translocation Down's syndrome." *Lancet* 1: 1191–93.

ROSS, J. D., MOLONEY, W. C., and DESFORGES, J. F. 1963. "Ineffective regulation of granulopoiesis masquerading as congenital leukemia in a mongoloid child." *J. Pediat.* 63: 1–10.

RUNDLE, A., COPPEN, A., and COWIE, V. 1961. "Steroid excretion in mothers of mongols." *Lancet* 2: 846–48.

RUNDEL, A. T., DUTTON, G., and GIBSON, J. 1959. "Endocrinological aspects of mental deficiency. I. Testicular function in mongolism." *J. Ment. Defic. Res.* 3: 108–15.

RUNGE, G. H. 1958–59. "Glucose tolerance in mongolism." *Amer. J. Ment. Defic.* 63: 822–28.

SANDRUCCI, M. G. and PICCOTTI, M. L. 1957. "La funzionalità cortico-surrenalica nel mongolismo." *Min. Pediat.* 9: 1368–72.

SAXENA, K. M. and PRYLES, C. V. 1965. "Thyroid function in mongolism." *J. Pediat.* 67: 363–70.

SCHERZ, R. G. 1962. "Negro female mongol with 46 chromosomes." *Lancet* 2: 882.

SCHMICKEL, R. 1967. "Chromosome aberrations in leukocytes exposed in vitro to diagnostic levels of X-rays." *Amer. J. Hum. Genet.* 19: 1–11.

SCHULL, W. J. and NEEL, J. V. 1962. "Maternal radiation and mongolism." *Lancet* 1: 537–38.

SCHUNK, G. J. and LEHMAN, W. L. 1954. "Mongolism and congenital leukemia." *J.A.M.A.* 155: 250–51.

SÉQUIN, É. 1846. "Traitement moral, hygiène et education des idiots et des autres enfants arrières ou retardes dans leur développement." Paris: J. B. Baillière. Cited in: *Progress in Medical Genetics,* 1964. vol. III. New York and London: Grune and Stratton.

SERGOVICH, F. R., SOLTAN, H. C., and CARR, D. H. 1964. "Twelve unrelated translocation mongols: Cytogenetic, genetics, and parental age data." *Cytogenetics* 3: 34–44.

SHAPIRO, A. 1949. "The differential leucocyte count in children with mongolism." *J. Ment. Sci.* 95: 689.

SHAPIRO, S., JONES, E. W., and DENSEN, P. M. 1962. "A life table of pregnancy termination and correlates of fetal loss." *Milbank Memorial Fund Quart.* 40: 7–45.

SHAW, M. W. 1962. "Familial mongolism." *Cytogenetics* 1: 141–79.

SHUTTLEWORTH, G. E. 1909. "Mongolian imbecility." *Brit. Med. J.* 2: 661–65.

SIGLER, A. T., COHEN, B. H., LILIENFELD, A. M., WESTLAKE, J. E., and HETZNECKER, W. H. 1967. "Reproductive and marital experience of parents of children with Down's syndrome (mongolism)." *J. Pediat.* 70: 608–14.

SIGLER, A. T., LILIENFELD, A. M., COHEN, B. H., and WESTLAKE, J. E. 1965*a*. "Radiation exposure of parents of children with mongolism (Down's syndrome)." *Bull. Johns Hopkins Hosp.* 117: 374–99.

———. 1965*b*. "Parental age in Down's syndrome (mongolism)." *J. Pediat.* 67: 631–42.

SIMON, A., LUDWIG, C., GOFMAN, J. W., and CROOK, G. H. 1954–55. "Metabolic studies in mongolism: Serum protein-bound iodine, cholesterol, and lipoprotein." *Amer. J. Psych.* 3: 139–45.

SKANSE, B. and LAURELL, C. B. 1962. "The immune-globulins in mongolism." *Acta Med. Scand.* 172: 63–65.

SLATER, B. C. S., WATSON, G. I., and McDONALD, J. C. 1964. "Seasonal variation in congenital abnormalities: Preliminary report of a survey conducted by the Research Committee of Council of the College of General Practitioners." *Brit. J. Prev. Soc. Med.* 18: 1–7.

SMITH, A. and RECORD, R. G. 1955*a*. "Maternal age and birth rank in the aetiology of mongolism." *Brit. J. Prev. Soc. Med.* 9: 51–55.

———. 1955*b*. "Fertility and reproductive history of mothers of mongoloid defectives." *Brit. J. Prev. Soc. Med.* 9: 89–96.

SMITH, G. F. 1964. "Mosaic mongols," in: *Proc. International Copenhagen Congress on the Scientific Study of Mental Retardation,* vol. 1, pp. 173–78.

SNELL, G. D. and PICKEN, D. I. 1935. "Abnormal development in the mouse caused by chromosome unbalance." *J. Genet.* 31: 213–35.

SOBEL, A. E., STRAZZULA, M., SHERMAN, B. S., ELKAN, B., MORGENSTERN, S. W., MARIUS, N., and MEISEL, A. 1957–58. "Vitamin A absorption and other blood composition studies in mongolism." *Amer. J. Ment. Defic.* 62: 642–56.

SPELLMAN, M. P. 1966. "Mongolism—Survey in Cork City and County." *J. Irish Med. Assoc.* 59: 12–13.

SPINELLI-RESSI, F. and BERGONZI, F. 1963. "Red cell triiodothyronine uptake as a measure of thyroid function in mongolism." *Acta Paed.* 52: 575–80.

STARK, C. R. 1963. "The occurrence of congenital anomalies and malignant neoplasms in a group of families containing a proband with Down's syndrome and in a group of matched control families." Thesis, Dr. P. H., University of Michigan.

STARK, C. R. and FRAUMENI, J. F., JR. 1966. "Viral hepatitis and Down's syndrome." *Lancet* 1: 1036–37.

STARK, C. R. and MANTEL, N. 1966. "Effects of maternal age and birth order on the risk of mongolism and leukemia." *J. Nat. Cancer Inst.* 37: 687–98.

———. 1967. "Lack of seasonal- or temporal-spatial clustering of Down's syndrome births in Michigan." *Amer. J. Epid.* 86: 199–213.

STARKMAN, M. N. and SHAW, M. W. 1967. "Atypical acrocentric chromosomes in Negro and Caucasian mongols." *Amer. J. Hum. Genet.* 19: 162–73.

STERN, J. 1965. "Biochemical aspects of Down's disease," in: *Biochemical Approaches to Mental Handicap in Children,* ed. J. D. ALLAN and K. S. HOLT, pp. 40–51. Baltimore: Williams & Wilkins Company.

STERN, J. and LEWIS, W. H. P. 1957*a*. "Serum proteins in mongolism." *J. Ment. Sci.* 103: 222–26.

———. 1957*b*. "The serum cholesterol level in children with mongolism and other mentally retarded children." *J. Ment. Defic. Res.* 1: 96–106.

———. 1958. "Calcium, phosphate and phosphatase in mongolism." *J. Ment. Sci.* 104: 880–83.

_______. 1959. "The serum lipoproteins of mentally retarded children." *J. Ment. Sci.* 105: 1012–16.

_______. 1959–60. "Blood magnesium in children with mongolism and other mentally retarded children." *Amer. J. Ment. Defic.* 64: 972–77.

_______. 1962. "Serum esterase in mongolism." *J. Ment. Defic. Res.* 6: 13–21.

STEVENSON, A.C., JOHNSTON, H. A., STEWART, M. I. P., and GOLDING, D. R. 1966. "Congenital malformations: A report of a study of series of consecutive births in 24 centres." *Bull. WHO,* Suppl., 34: 9–127.

STEVENSON, S. S., WORCESTER, J., and RICE, R. G. 1950. "677 congenitally malformed infants and associated gestational characteristics." *Pediatrics* 6: 37–50.

STEWART, A., WEBB, J., and HEWITT, D. 1958. "A survey of childhood malignancies." *Brit. Med. J.* 1: 1495–1508.

STOLLER, A. and COLLMANN, R. D. 1965*a*. "Incidence of infective hepatitis followed by Down's syndrome nine months later." *Lancet* 2: 1221–23.

_______. 1965*b*. "Patterns of occurrence of births in Victoria, Australia, producing Down's syndrome (mongolism) and congenital anomalies of the central nervous system: A 21-year prospective and retrospective survey." *Med. J. Aust.* 1: 1–4.

_______. 1965*c*. "Virus aetiology for Down's syndrome (mongolism)." *Nature* 208: 903–04.

_______. 1966. "Area relationship between incidences of infectious hepatitis and of the births of children with Down's syndrome nine months later." *J. Ment. Defic. Res.* 10: 84–88.

STOTT, D. H. 1961. "Mongolism related to emotional shock in early pregnancy." *Vita Humana* 4: 57–76.

STURTEVANT, A. H. 1929. "The 'claret' mutant type of drosophilia simulans: A study of chromosome elimination and of cell lineage." *Z. Wiss. Zool.* 135: 323–56.

SUGIYAMA, T., KURITA, Y., and NISHIZUKA, Y. 1967. "Chromosome abnormality in rat leukemia induced by 7, 12-dimethylbenz [a] anthracene." *Science* 158: 1058–59.

SZULMAN, A. E. 1965. "Chromosomal aberrations in spontaneous human abortions." *New Eng. J. Med.* 272: 811–18.

THIEDE, H. A. and SALM, S. B. 1964. "Chromosome studies of human spontaneous abortions." *Amer. J. Obstet. Gynec.* 90: 205–15.

TOMPKINS, A. B. 1964. "Down's syndrome in Nigerian children." *J. Med. Genet.* 1: 115–17.

TONOMURA, A., OISHI, H., MATSUNAGA, E., and KURITA, T. 1966. "Down's syndrome: A cytogenetic and statistical survey of 127 Japanese patients." *Jap. J. Hum. Genet.* 11: 1–16.

TRICOMI, V., VALENTI, C., and HALL, J. E. 1964. "Ovulatory patterns in Down's syndrome." *Amer. J. Obstet. Gynec.* 89: 651–56.

TRUBOWITZ, S., KIRMAN, D., and MASEK, B. 1962. "The leucocyte alkaline phosphatase in mongolism." *Lancet* 2: 486–87.

TURNER, J. H. 1962. "The mongoloid phenotype: Its incidence, etiology and association with leukemia and other neoplastic disease." Thesis, Sc.D., Hyg., University of Pittsburgh.

———. 1963. "Mongolism (Down's syndrome): Prevalence, sex distribution and mortality." *Penn. Psych. Quart.,* (Summer issue): 3–21.

TURPIN, R. and BERNYER, G. 1947. "De l'influence de l'hérédité sur la formule D'Arneth (cas particulier du mongolisme)." *Rev. Hemat.* 2: 190–206.

UCHIDA, I. A. and CURTIS, E. J. 1961. "A possible association between maternal radiation and mongolism." *Lancet* 2: 848–50.

U.S. DEPARTMENT OF HEALTH, EDUCATION AND WELFARE. 1962. Public Health Service. Vital Statistics of the United States, 1960, vol. 1, *Natality.* Washington: U.S. Government Printing Office.

WAARDENBURG, P. J. 1932. "Mongolismus: Das menschliche auge und seine erbanlagen." *Biobio. Genet.* 7: 44–48. The Hague-Nijhoff.

WALD, N., BORGES, W. H., LI, C. C., TURNER, J. H., and HARNOIS, M. C. 1961. "Leukaemia associated with mongolism." *Lancet* 1: 1228.

WALKER, N. F., CARR, D. H., SERGOVICH, F. R., BARR, M. L., and SOLTAN, H. C. 1963. "Trisomy-21 and 13-15/21 translocation chromosome patterns in related mongol defectives." *J. Ment. Defic. Res.* 7: 150–63.

WAXMAN, S. H., ARAKAKI, M. S., and SMITH, J. B. 1967. "Cytogenetics of fetal abortions." *Pediatrics* 39: 425–32.

WEGELIUS, R., VÄÄNÄNEN, I., and KOSKELA, S.-L. 1967. "Down's syndrome and transient leukaemia-like disease in a newborn." *Acta Paed. Scand.* 56: 301–06.

WEINSTEIN, E. D., RUCKNAGEL, D. L., and SHAW, M. W. 1965. "Quantitative studies on A_2, sickle cell, and fetal hemoglobins in Negroes with mongolism, with observations on translocation mongolism in Negroes." *Amer. J. Hum. Genet.* 17: 443–56.

WILTON, E. 1964. "Chromosome investigation of Bantu and coloured patients with the Langdon-Down syndrome." *Med. Proc.* 10: 171–76.

WORLD HEALTH ORGANIZATION STUDY GROUP. 1966. Geneva Conference. "Standardization of procedures for chromosome studies in abortion." *Cytogenetics* 5: 361–93.

WRIGHT, S. W., DAY, R. W., MOSIER, H. D., KOONS, A., and MUELLER, H. 1963. "Klinefelter's syndrome, Down's syndrome (mongolism), and twinning in the same sibship." *J. Pediat.* 62: 217–24.

WRIGHT, S. W., DAY, R. W., MULLER, H., and WEINHOUSE, R. 1967. "The frequency of trisomy and translocation in Down's syndrome." *J. Pediat.* 70: 420–24.

WRIGHT, S. W. and FINK, K. 1957. "The excretion of beta-aminoisobutyric acid in normal, mongoloid and non-mongoloid mentally defective children." *Amer. J. Ment. Defic.* 61: 530–33.

YOKOYAMA, M. 1966. "Immunogenetic studies on mongolism." *Hawaii Med.* J. 26: 121–24.

ZELLWEGER, H. 1964. "Familial mongolism: History and present status." *Clin. Pediat.* 3: 291–303.

Selected Bibliography

AARSKOG, D. 1966. "A new cytogenetic variant of translocation Down's syndrome." *Cytogenetics* 5: 82–87.

AGNOSTO, D. 1948. "Observations on the fate of children with mongolism." *Clin. Pediat.* 30: 131–35.

ÅKESSON, H. O. 1963. "Urban-rural distribution of low-grade mental defectives." *Acta Genet.* 13: 275–89.

ALLEN, G. and KALLMANN, F. J. 1955. "Frequency and types of mental retardation in twins." *Amer. J. Hum. Genet.* 7: 15–20.

BARKER, D. J. P. and RECORD, R. G. 1967. "The relationship of the presence of disease to birth order and maternal age." *Amer. J. Hum. Genet.* 19: 433–49.

BEALL, G. and STANTON, R. G. 1945. "Reduction in the number of mongolian defectives—A result of family limitation." *Canad. J. Public Health* 36: 33–37.

BELLING, J. 1933. "Crossing over and gene rearrangement in flowering plants." *Genetics* 18: 387–413.

BENDA, C. E. 1951. "Empiric risk figures in mongolism." *Amer. J. Ment. Defic.* 55: 539–45.

————. 1959. "Mongolism: Clinical manifestations, pathology and etiology," in: *Proc. First International Conference on Mental Retardation,* ed. P. W. BOWMAN and H. V. MOUTNER, pp. 340–63.

————. 1965. "Mongolism," in: *Medical Aspects of Mental Retardation,* pp. 519–90. Springfield, Ill.: Charles C Thomas.

BENYESH-MELNICK, M., STICH, H. F., RAPP, F., and HSU, T. C. 1964. "Viruses and mammalian chromosomes. III. Effect of herpes zoster virus on human embryonal lung cultures." *Proc. Soc. Exp. Biol. Med.* 117: 546–49.

BEOLCHINI, P. E. 1964. "Ricerche statistiche e genetiche sulle malformazioni congenite." *Acta Gen. Med. Gemell.* 13: 203–15.

BISHOP, K. and CONNOLLY, J. M. 1965. "Chromosomes and mental retardation," in: *Medical Aspects of Mental Retardation.* Springfield, Ill.: Charles C Thomas.

BLATTNER, R. J. 1961. "Chromosomes in chronic myeloid leukemia and in acute leukemia associated with mongolism." *J. Pediat.* 59: 145–48.

BLEYER, A. 1932. "The frequency of mongoloid imbecility: The question of race and the apparent influence of sex." *Amer. J. Dis. Child.* 44: 503–08.

———. 1938. "Role of advanced maternal age in causing mongolism: A study of 2,822 cases." *Amer. J. Dis. Child.* 55: 79–92.

BODMER, W. F. 1961. "Effects of maternal age on the incidence of congenital abnormalities in mouse and man." *Nature* 190: 1134–35.

BRAIN, L. 1967. "Chairman's opening remarks: Historical introduction," in: Ciba Foundation Study Group No. 25, *Mongolism,* pp. 1–5. Boston: Little, Brown and Company.

BRANDT, N. J. 1963. "Galactose-1-phosphate-uridyl-transferase in oligophrenic patients: With special reference to patients with Down's syndrome." *Dan. Med. Bull.* 10: 50–51.

BREG, W. R., CORNWELL, J. G., and MILLER, O. J. 1962. "The association of the triple-X syndrome and mongolism in two families." *Amer. J. Dis. Child.* 104: 534–35.

BRIDGES, C. B. 1929. "Variation in crossing over in relation to age of female in drosophila melanogaster," in: STURTEVANT, A. H., BRIDGES, C. B., MORGAN, T. H., MORGAN, L. V., and LI, J. C. *Contributions to the Genetics of Drosophila Stimulans and Drosophila Melanogaster.* Carnegie Institution of Washington, Pub. No. 399, pp. 65–89.

BURCH, P. R. J., ROWELL, N. R., and BURWELL, R. G. 1966. "Autoimmunity and chromosomal aberrations." *Lancet* 2: 170.

CARR, D. H. 1962. "The chromosome abnormality in mongolism." *Canad. Med. Assoc. J.* 87: 490–95.

CHRISTIE, A. and GLADISH, M. L. 1966. "Origin of the terms 'mongolism' and 'Down's syndrome'. " *J. Pediat.* 68: 675–76.

CHU, E. H. Y., RUBINSTEIN, J. H., and WARKANY, J. 1961. "Chromosome studies in a family with four cases of atypical Down's syndrome." *Proc. Second International Congress on Human Genetics* 2: 1169–75.

CLARKE, C. A. 1964. "The chromosomes of man," in: *Genetics for the Clinician* (second edition), pp. 14–39. Philadelphia: F. A. Davis Co.

COHEN, B. H., LILIENFELD, A. M., and SIGLER, A. T. 1963. "Some epidemiological aspects of mongolism: A review." *Amer. J. Public Health* 53: 223–36.

COHEN, M. M. and DAVIDSON, R. G. 1967. "Down's syndrome associated with a familial (21q −; 22q +) translocation." *Cytogenetics* 6: 321–30.

COLLMANN, R. D. and STOLLER, A. 1962. "Epidemiology of congenital anomalies of the central nervous system with special reference to patterns in the State of Victoria, Australia." *J. Ment. Defic. Res.* 6: 22–37.

———. 1963. "Data on mongolism in Victoria, Australia: Prevalence and life expectation." *J. Ment. Defic. Res.* 7: 60–68.

CONEN, P. E., BELL, A. G., and RANCE, C. P. 1962. "A review of chromosome studies in the diagnosis of mongolism." *J. Pediat.* 60: 533–39.

CONEN, P. E. and ERKMAN, B. 1966. "Combined mongolism and leukemia." *Amer. J. Dis. Child.* 112: 429–43.

COOKE, J. V. 1954. "The occurrence of leukemia." *Blood* 9: 340–47.

CROSS, H. E. and MCKUSICK, V. A. 1966. "Mongolism in an inbred population." *Bull. Johns Hopkins Hosp.* 119: 268–75.

DAWSON, W. R. 1909. "Considerations upon the report of the Royal Commission on the care and control of the feeble-minded." *Brit. Med. J.* 2: 665–69.

DAY, R. W. 1964. "Completeness of birth certificate reporting for mongolism (Down's syndrome)." *Public Health Rep.* 79: 19–24.

DEGALÁN, E. H. K. 1966. "Genetics: Age and chromosomes." *Nature* 211: 1324–25.

DENT, T., EDWARDS, J. H.. and DELHANTY, J. D. A. 1963. "A partial mongol." *Lancet* 2: 484–87.

EL-ALFI, O. S., SMITH, P. M. and BIESELE, J. J. 1965. "Chromosomal breaks in human leucocyte cultures induced by an agent in the plasma of infectious hepatitis patients." *Hereditas* 52: 285–94.

ENGLER, M. 1952. "A comparative study of the causation of mongolism, peristatic amentia, and other types of mental defect." *J. Ment. Sci.* 98: 316–25.

EVANS, D. A. P., DONOHOE, W. T. A., BANNERMAN, R. M., MOHN, J. F., and LAMBERT, R. M. 1966. "Blood-group gene localization through a study of mongolism." *Ann. Hum. Genet.* 30: 49–67.

FEDERMAN, D. D., SHANNON, D. C., CRAWFORD, J. D., DODGE, P. R., and CONNELLY, J. P. 1965. "Down's syndrome." *Clin. Pediat.* 4: 331–41.

FIALKOW, P. J. 1964. "Autoimmunity: A predisposing factor to chromosomal aberrations?" *Lancet* 1: 474–75.

FISCHER, R., GRIFFIN, F., and KAPLAN, A. R. 1962. "Taste thresholds in mothers of children with Down's syndrome." *Lancet* 2: 992.

FISCHER, R., GRIFFIN, F., ENGLAND, S., and PASAMANICK, B. 1961. "Biochemical-genetic factors of taste-polymorphism and their relation to salivary thyroid metabolism in health and mental retardation." *Med. Exp.* 4: 356–66.

FRACCARO, M., KAIJSER, K., and LINDSTEN, J. 1960. "Chromosomal abnormalities in father and mongol child." *Lancet* 1: 724–27.

FRAUMENI, J. F., JR., and LUNDIN, F. E., JR. 1966. "Infective hepatitis and Down's syndrome." *Lancet* 1: 712–13.

FRIEDMAN, A. 1955. "Mongolism in twins." *Amer. J. Dis. Child.* 90: 43–50.

GIANNELLI, F., HAMERTON, J. L., and CARTER, C. O. 1965. "Cytogenetics of Down's syndrome (mongolism) II. The frequency of interchange trisomy in patients born at a maternal age of less than 30 years." *Cytogenetics* 4: 186–92.

GIRALDO, G., RIBACCHI, R., and BOLLOLI, D. 1966. "On the possible association between maternal viral hepatitis and Down's syndrome." *Lav. Anat. Pat. Perugia* 26: 15–28.

GLANVILLE, E. V. 1964. "Mongolism: A clue to the source of the accessory chromosome?" *Lancet* 2: 1065–66.

GOLDMAN, A. S. 1965. "Predisposing genetic and metabolic factors to developmental defects of the central nervous system." *J. Amer. Phys. Ther. Assoc.* 45: 345–56.

GOODLIN, R. C. 1965. "Non-disjunction and maternal age in the mouse." *J. Reprod. Fertil.* 9: 355–56.

GOODMAN, H. O., KING, J. S., and THOMAS, J. J. 1964. "Urinary excretion of beta-amino-isobutyric acid and taurine in mongolism." *Nature* 204: 650–52.

GOODMAN, H. O. and THOMAS, J. J. 1966. "ABO frequencies in mongolism." *Ann. Hum. Genet.* 30: 43–48.

GOODMAN, N. and TIZARD, J. 1962. "Prevalence of imbecility and idiocy among children." *Brit. Med. J.* 1: 216–19.

GREENBERG, R. C. 1964. "Some factors in the epidemiology of mongolism," in: *Proc. International Copenhagen Congress on the Scientific Study of Mental Retardation (2nd Conf.),* vol. 1, pp. 200–02.

GUSTAVSON, K. H. 1961. "Chromosomal abnormality in a mongolism-like syndrome." *Proc. Second International Congress on Human Genetics* 2: 1179–81.

HALL, B. 1962. "Down's syndrome (mongolism) with normal chromosomes." *Lancet* 2: 1026–27.

———. 1964. "Mongolism-fetalism." *Proc. International Copenhagen Congress on the Scientific Study of Mental Retardation,* vol. 1, pp. 203–06.

———. 1966. "Mongolism in newborn infants: An examination of the criteria for recognition and some speculations on the pathogenic activity of the chromosomal abnormality." *Clin. Pediat.* 5: 4–12.

HAMERTON, J. L., COWIE, V. A., GIANNELLI, F., BRIGGS, S. M., and POLANI, P. E. 1961. "Differential transmission of Down's syndrome (mongolism) through male and female translocation carriers." *Lancet* 2: 956–58.

HAMPAR, B. and ELLISON, S. A. 1961. "Chromosomal aberrations induced by an animal virus." *Nature* 192: 145–47.

HARD, W. L., EISEN, J. D., and STANAGE, W. F. 1965. "The familial transmission of G/G chromosome in a case of Down's syndrome." *S. Dakota Med. J.* 18: 15–17.

HARNDEN, D. G. 1961. "The chromosomes," in: PENROSE, L. S. *Recent Advances in Human Genetics,* pp. 19–38. Boston: Little, Brown and Company.

HASSAN, M. M. 1962. "Mongolism in Sudanese children." *J. Trop. Pediat. African Child Health* 8: 48–50.

HECHT, F., BRYANT, J. S., GRUBER, D., and TOWNES, P. L. 1964. "The nonrandomness of chromosomal abnormalities: Association of trisomy 18 and Down's syndrome." *New Eng. J. Med.* 271: 1081–86.

HELD, A. J. and HURNY, J. 1966. "Fluorides and mongolism." *Schweiz. Mschr. Zahnheilk* 76: 607–09.

HIENZ, H. A. 1965. "Zur cytogenetik des mongolismus unter besonderer berücksichtigung der familiären form." *Verh. d. Dtsch. Ges. f. Path.* 49: 333–38.

HIRSCHHORN, K., COOPER, H. L., MEYER, L. M., SKLARIN, B. S., and RENDON, O. R. 1961. "A case of mongolism with chromosomal translocation, familial giant satellites and leukemia." *Proc. Second International Congress on Human Genetics* 2: 1183–86.

HOLT, S. B. 1961. "Current advances in our knowledge of the inheritance of variations in finger-prints." *Proc. Second International Congress on Human Genetics* 3: 1450–57.

HUNGERFORD, D. A. 1964. "The Philadelphia chromosome and some others." *Ann. Int. Med.* 61: 789–93.

INGALLS, T. H. and KLINGBERG, M. A. 1965. "Congenital malformations: Clinical and community considerations." *Amer. J. Med. Sci.* 249: 104–32.

IRWIN, J. O. 1965. "A theory of the association (overlap) of chromosomes in karyotypes, illustrated by Dr. Patrica Jacobs' data." *Ann. Hum. Genet.* 28: 361–67.

JARVIK, L. F. 1963. "Senescence and chromosomal changes." *Lancet* 1: 114–15.

JARVIK, L. F., FALEK, A., and PIERSON, W. P. 1964. "Down's syndrome (mongolism): The heritable aspects." *Psych. Bull.* 61: 388–98.

JELLIFFE, D. B. 1954. "Mongolism in Jamaican children." *W. Indian Med. J.* 3: 164–65.

JERVIS, G. A. 1943. "Mongolism in twins." *Amer. J. Ment. Defic.* 47: 364–69.

JOHNSTON, A. W. 1961. "The familial occurrence of chromosome abnormalities." *Proc. Second International Congress on Human Genetics* 2: 1191–93.

JOHNSTON, A. W. and PETRAKIS. J. K. 1963. "Mongolism and Turner's syndrome in the same sibship." *Ann. Hum. Genet.* 26: 407–13.

KAPLAN, A. R. and ZSAKO, S. 1966. "Down's syndrome associated with family history of malignancy in mothers of affected children." *Amer. J. Ment. Defic.* 70: 866–72.

KOENIG, E. U., LUBS, H. A., JR., and BRANDT, I. K. 1962. "The relationship between congenital anomalies and autosomal chromosome abnormalities." *Yale J. Biol. Med.* 35: 189–205.

KREHBIEL, E. L. 1966. "An estimation of the cumulative mutation rate for sex-linked lethals in man which produce fetal deaths." *Amer. J. Hum. Genet.* 18: 127–43.

KRIVIT, W. and GOOD, R. A. 1956. "The simultaneous occurrence of leukemia and mongolism: Report of four cases." *A.M.A. J. Dis. Child.* 91: 218–22.

KUSHNICK, T. 1961. "Mongolism: Recent studies and developments." *Quart. Rev. Pediat.* 16: 150–59.

LASHOF, J. C. and STEWART, A. 1965. "Oxford survey of childhood cancers: Progress report III: Leukaemia and Down's syndrome." *Monthly Bull. Minist. Health* 24: 136–43.

LASSEN, N. A., CHRISTENSEN, S., HOEDT-RASMUSSEN, K., and STEWART, B. M. 1966. "Cerebral oxygen consumption in Down's syndrome." *Arch. Neurol.* 15: 595–602.

LAZAR, M. 1953. "Mongolism." *Psych. Quart. Suppl.,* Part 2, pp. 1–10.

LEE, C. H. and CINER, E. 1957. "Congenital leukemia associated with mongolism: Report of a case." *J. Pediat.* 51: 303–05.

LEHMANN, O., FORSSMAN, H. and HÄLLSTRÖM, T. 1962. "Chromosome studies of persons with mongolism (Down's syndrome) born to young mothers." *Acta Soc. Med. Upsal.* 67: 285–89.

LEJEUNE, J. 1963. "Autosomal disorders." *Pediatrics* 32: 326–37.

LENZ, V. W., PFEIFFER, R. A., and TÜNTE, W. 1966. "Chromosomenanomalien durch überzahl (trisomien) und alter der mutter." *Dtsch. Med. Wschr.* 91: 1262–67.

LEWIS, E. B. and GENCARELLA, W. 1952. "Claret and non-disjunction in drosophila melanogaster." *Genetics* 37: 600–01.

LINDSTEN, J. 1963. "The nature and origin of X chromosome aberrations in Turner's syndrome: A cytogenetical and clinical study of 57 patients." pp. 9–167. Uppsala: Almqvist and Wiksell.

LUBS, H. A., JR., KOENIG, E. U., and BRANDT, I. K. 1961. "Trisomy 13–15: A clinical syndrome." *Lancet* 2: 1001–02.

LUDER, J. and MUSOKE, L. K. 1955. "Mongolism in Africans." *Arch. Dis. Child.* 30: 310–15.

MACLEAN, N., HARNDEN, D. G., and COURT-BROWN, W. M. 1961. "Abnormalities of sex chromosome constitution in newborn babies." *Lancet* 2: 406–08.

MACMAHON, B. and GORDON, J. E. 1953. "Epidemiologic inferences derived from maternal age." *Amer. J. Med. Sci.* 226: 326–49.

MALZBERG, B. 1950. "Some statistical aspects of mongolism." *Amer. J. Ment. Defic.* 54: 266–81.

MARSDEN, H. B., MACKAY, R. I., MURRAY, A., and WARD, H. E. 1966. "Down's syndrome with a familial D/D reciprocal translocation and a G/G chromosome." *J. Med. Genet.* 3: 56–58.

MATSUNAGA, E. 1964. "Vergleichende erbbiologie und erbpathologie von Europaern und Japanern." *Homo.* 15: 129–37.

McDONALD, A. D. 1964. "Mongolism in twins." *J. Med. Genet.* 1: 39–41.

MIKULOWSKI, V. 1960. "The problem of simultaneous occurrence of leukemia and mongolism." *Ann. Paed.* 195: 49–56.

MIKULOWSKI, W. 1959. "Bialaczka w mongolowatości." *Pol. Tyg. Lek.* 14: 2186–88.

MITTWOCH, U. 1958. "The polymorphonuclear lobe count in mongolism and its relation to the total leucocyte count." *J. Ment. Defic. Res.* 2: 75–80.

———. 1959. "The relationship between the leucocyte count, the 'shift to the left' and the incidence of drumsticks in mongolism." *Acta Genet., Med. Gemell. Suppl.,* 2: 131–38.

———. 1964. "Frequency of drumsticks in normal women and in patients with chromosomal abnormalities." *Nature* 201: 317–19.

———. 1964. "Sex chromatin." *J. Med. Genet.* 1: 50–76.

MONTAGU, M. F. A. 1963. "Environmental factors in genetic disease." *Arch. Environ. Health* 6: 651–55.

MOORE, M. K. and ENGEL, E. 1968. "G. chromosome trisomy: Five cases with syndromes other than classical Down's." *South. Med. J.* 61: 146–54.

MOORHEAD, P. S. and SAKSELA, E. 1965. "The sequence of chromosome aberrations during SV 40 transformation of a human diploid cell strain." *Hereditas* 52: 271–84.

MOSIER, H. D., SCOTT, L. W., and COTTER, L. H. 1960. "The frequency of the positive sex-chromatin pattern in males with mental deficiency." *Pediatrics* 25: 291–97.

MOTTRAM, J. C. 1930. "The effect of carbon dioxide on the occurrence of non-disjunction in drosophila." *J. Exper. Biol.* 7: 370–72.

MOTULSKY, A. G. and HECHT, F. 1964. "Genetic prognosis and counseling." *Amer. J. Obstet. Gynec.* 90: 1227–41.

MYERS, C. R. 1938. "An application of the control group method to the problem of the etiology of mongolism." *Proc. Amer. Assoc. Ment. Defic.* 43: 142–50.

NAEYE, R. L. 1967. "Prenatal organ and cellular growth with various chromosomal disorders." *Biol. Neonat.* 11: 248–60.

NICHOLS, W. W., LEVAN, A., AULA, P., and NORRBY, E. 1965. "Chromosome damage associated with the measles virus in vitro." *Hereditas* 54: 101–18.

NICHOLS, W. W., LEVAN, A., HENEEN, W. K., and PELUSE, M. 1965. "Synergism of the Schmidt-Ruppin strain of the rous sarcoma virus and cytidine triphosphate in the induction of chromosome breaks in human cultured leukocytes." *Hereditas* 54: 213–36.

PABST, H. F., PUESCHEL, S., and HILLMAN, D. A. 1967. "Etiologic interrelationship in Down's syndrome, hypothyroidism, and precocious sexual development." *Pediatrics* 40: 590–95.

PANIZON, F. 1965. "Neonatal jaundice in Down's syndrome." *Lancet* 2: 495.

PARSONS, P. A. 1964. "Parental age and the offspring." *Quart. Rev. Biol.* 39: 258–75.

PENROSE, L. S. 1933. "The relative effects of paternal and maternal age in mongolism." *J. Genet.* 27: 219–24.

———. 1951. "Maternal age in familial mongolism." *J. Ment. Sci.* 97: 738–47.

———. 1960. "Genetic causes of malformation and the search for their origins," in: *Ciba Foundation Symposium on Congenital Malformations,* ed. G. E. W. WOLSTENHOLME and C. M. O'CONNOR, pp. 22–31. Boston: Little, Brown and Company.

———. 1961. "Mongolism." *Brit. Med. Bull.* 17: 184–89.

———. 1964. "Genetical aspects of mental deficiency," in: *Proc. International Copenhagen Congress on the Scientific Study of Mental Retardation (2nd Conf.)*, vol. 1, p. 165.

———. 1965. "Dermatoglyphics in mosaic mongolism and allied conditions," in: *Genetics Today,* ed. S. J. GEERTS, pp. 973–80. Oxford: Pergamon Press.

PHILLPOTTS, J. S. 1966. "Radiation and mongolism." *Lancet* 1: 1324.

PITT, D. 1965. "Recurrence risks in mental deficiency." *Med. J. Aust.* 2: 184–87.

POLANI, P. E. 1962. "Mongolism." *J. Obstet. Gynec.* 69: 822–30.

———. 1966. "Chromosome anomalies and abortions." *Develop. Med. Child Neurol.* 8: 67–70.

POWARS, D., ROHDE, R., and GRAVES, D. 1964. "Foetal haemoglobin and neutrophil anomaly in the D_1-trisomy syndrome." *Lancet* 1: 1363–64.

RAY, S. D. 1964. "Some aetiological factors in mongolism observed in New Delhi." *J. Indian Med. Assoc.* 42: 15–17.

RECORD, R. G. and MCKEOWN, T. 1949. "Distribution of malformations and controls in the same maternal age groups at different birth ranks." *Brit. J. Soc. Med.* 3: 202–06.

REES, H. and NAYLOR, B. 1960. "Developmental variation in chromosome behaviour." *Heredity* 15: 17–27.

RENKONEN, K. O. 1966. "The birth of mongoloids." *Acta Genet.* 16: 276–82.

RENKONEN, K. O. and DONNER, M. 1964. "Mongoloids, their mothers and sibships." *Ann. Med. Exp. Fenn.* 42: 139–44.

———. 1965. "Mongoloids, twins and tolerance." *Ann. Med. Exp. Fenn.* 43: 215–22.

———. 1965. "The sibships posterior to mongoloids." *Ann. Med. Exp. Fenn.* 43: 72–81.

RENWICK, D. H. G. 1967. "Estimating prevalence of certain chronic childhood conditions by use of a central registry." *Public Health Rep.* 82: 261–69.

RICHARDS, B. W. 1964. "New work on Down's syndrome (mongolism): A review of the recent literature." *Develop. Med. Child Neurol.* 6: 175–82.

RIDLER, M. A. C. and SHAPIRO, A. 1959. "The longitudinal study of the leucocyte count in infants with mongolism." *J. Ment. Defic. Res.* 9:96–102.

ROBERTSON, J., MELLON, J. P., and STEWART, J. S. 1965. "Down's syndrome with unusual karyotype and thyroid autoantibodies." *J. Ment. Defic. Res.* 9: 157–63.

ROBINSON, A. 1961. "The human chromosomes." *Amer. J. Dis. Child.* 101: 133–52.

ROBINSON, A. and PUCK, T. T. 1965. "Sex chromatin in newborns: Presumptive evidence for external factors in human non-disjunction." *Science* 148: 83–85.

———. 1966. "Infective hepatitis and Down's syndrome." *Lancet* 1: 313–14.

ROHDE, R. and BERMAN, N. 1963. "The Lyon hypothesis and further malformation postulates in the chromosomal syndromes." *Lancet* 2: 1169–70.

ROSENKRANZ, V. W., FALK, W., PICHLER, A., and WASCHER, H. 1964. "Familiäres vorkommen von chromosomenaberrationen." *Helv. Paed. Acta* 19: 444–57.

ROSNER, F., ONG, B. H., MAHANAND, D., PAINE, R. S., and JACOBSON, C. B. 1964. "Leucocyte enzymes in Down's syndrome." *Lancet* 2: 1345–46.

ROWE, R. D. and UCHIDA, I. A. 1961. "Cardiac malformation in mongolism: A prospective study of 184 mongoloid children." *Amer. J. Med.* 31: 726–35.

ROWLEY, J. D. 1961–62. "A review of recent studies of chromosomes in mongolism." *Amer. J. Ment. Defic.* 66: 529–32.

RUGH, R. and WOHLFROMM, M. 1963. "Age of the mother and previous breeding history and the incidence of X-ray induced congenital anomalies." *Radiat. Res.* 19: 261–69.

RYAN, J. P. A. 1964. "The incidence of cardiac abnormalities in mongolism." *Proc. International Copenhagen Congress on the Scientific Study of Mental Retardation,* vol. 1, pp. 215–17.

SAKSELA, E., AULA, P., and CANTELL, K. 1965. "Chromosomal damage of human cells induced by Sendai virus." *Ann. Med. Exp. Fenn.* 43: 132–36.

SARIN, B. P. 1960. "Mongolism in children of Mongolian races." *Burma Med. J.* 8: 4–7.

SCHACHTER, M. 1961. "Mongolisme et race: À propos d'une fillette mongolienne de race noire." *J. Génét. Hum.* 10: 202–09.

SCHADE, H. 1963. "Chromosomenanomalien beim menschen (III) eine übersicht." *Med. Welt.* 51: 2593–99.

SERGOVICH, F. R., LUCE, A., and CARR, D. H. 1967. "Chromosome aneuploidy in the father of a mongol." *Amer. J. Dis. Child.* 114: 407–11.

SHAPIRO, A. 1963. "The importance of chromosome studies in relation to mental deficiency" in: *Proc. Second International Congress on Mental Retardation, Vienna, 1961,* Part I, pp. 346–52.

SHAW, M. W. 1962. "Segregation ratios and linkage studies in a family with six translocation mongols." *Lancet* 1: 1407.

SHAW, M. W. and GERSHOWITZ, H. 1962. "A search for autosomal linkage in a trisomic population: Blood group frequencies in mongols." *Amer. J. Hum. Genet.* 14: 317–34.

———. 1963. "Blood group frequencies in mongols." *Amer. J. Hum. Genet.* 15: 495–96.

SHETTY, K. T., SHARMA, N. L., and WAHAL, K. M. 1966. "Mongolism, leukemia and sex chromatin anomalies." *Indian J. Pediat.* 33: 103–06.

SLIZYNSKI, B. M. 1960. "Sexual dimorphism in mouse gametogenesis." *Genet. Res.* 1: 477–86.

———. 1961. "The Pachytene stage in mammalian oocytes." *Nature* 189: 683–84.

SMITH, D. W. 1964. "Autosomal abnormalities." *Amer. J. Obstet. Gynec.* 90: 1055–77.

SMITH, G. F., PENROSE, L. S., and O'HARA, P. T. 1967. "Crystalline bodies in lymphocytes of patients with Down's syndrome." *Lancet* 2: 452–53.

SOLTAN, H. C., WEINS, R. G., and SERGOVICH, F. R. 1964. "Genetic studies and chromosomal analyses in families with mongolism (Down's syndrome) in more than one member." *Acta Genet.* (Basel) 14: 251–64.

SOUDEK, D., LAXOVÁ, R., and ADAMEK, R. 1966. "Development of translocation 21/22." *Lancet* 2: 336–37.

STEWART, A. and HEWITT, D. 1965. "Leukaemia incidence in children in relation to radiation exposure in early life," in: *Current Topics in Radiation Research,* vol. 1, pp. 223–53. Amsterdam: North-Holland Publishing Company.

STICH, H. F., VAN HOOSIER, G. L., and TRENTIN, J. J. 1964. "Viruses and mammalian chromosomes." *Exper. Cell Res.* 34: 400–03.

STILES, K. A. and GOODMAN, H. O. 1961. "Reproduction in mongoloids," in: *Proc. Second International Congress on Human Genetics,* vol. 3.

STIMSON, C. W. 1967. "Translocation and familial mongolism." *Mich. Med.* 66: 1255–58.

STOLLER, A. 1961. "Investigation of mental deficiency." *Med. J. Aust.* 2: 206–10.

STOLLER, A. and COLLMANN, R. D. 1964. "Further observations on an infective hypothesis for the origin of mongolism and congenital anomalies of the central nervous system," in: *Proc. International Copenhagen Congress on the Scientific Study of Mental Retardation (2nd Conf.),* vol. 1, pp. 218–23.

———. 1966. "Viral hepatitis and Down's syndrome." *Lancet* 2: 339.

STORTS, B. P. 1956. "Mongolism and acute leukemia: A case report." *Ariz. Med.* 13: 408–09.

TAN, G. and SENG, C. T. 1966. "Familial mongolism—with leukaemia in one member and a normal twinsib in another." *J. Singapore Paed. Soc.* 8: 90–95.

THOMPSON, H. 1965. "Abnormalities of the autosomal chromosomes associated with human disease: Selected topics and catalogue." *Amer. J. Med. Sci.* 250: 140–56.

TOUGH, I. M., BAIKIE, A. G., HARNDEN, D. G., KING, M. J., COURT-BROWN, W. M., BUCKTON, K. E., JACOBS, P. A., and MCBRIDE, J. A. 1961. "Cytogenetic studies in chronic myeloid leukaemia and acute leukaemia associated with mongolism." *Lancet* 1: 411–17.

TOWNES, P. L., DEHART, K. G., JR., and ZIEGLER, N. A. 1964. "Trisomy 17–18—An evaluation of preconceptional parental irradiation as a possible etiologic factor." *J. Pediat.* 65: 870–79.

TSUANG, M. T. and LIN, T. Y. 1964. "A clinical and family study of Chinese mongol children." *J. Ment. Defic. Res.* 8: 84–91.

TUMPEER, I. H. 1922. "Mongolian idiocy in a Chinese boy." *J.A.M.A.* 79: 14–16.

WAGNER, H. R. 1962. "Mongolism in Orientals." *Amer. J. Dis. Child.* 103: 112–20.

WARBURTON, D. and FRASER, F. C. 1964. "Spontaneous abortion risks in man: Data from reproductive histories collected in a medical genetics unit." *Hum. Genet.* 16: 1–25.

WARKANY, J. 1960. "Etiology of mongolism." *J. Pediat.* 56: 412–19.

WARKANY, J., WEINSTEIN, E. D., SOUKUP, S. W., RUBINSTEIN, J. H., and CURLESS, M. C. 1964. "Chromosome analyses in a children's hospital: Selection of patients and results of studies." *Pediatrics* 33: 454–65.

WARNER, E. N. 1935. "A survey of mongolism, with a review of one hundred cases." *Canad. Med. Assoc. J.* 33: 495–500.

WAXMAN, S. H. and ARAKAKI, D. T. 1966. "Familial mongolism by a G/G mosaic carrier." *J. Pediat.* 69: 274–78.

WOOLF, C. M. 1965. "Stillbirths and parental age." *Obstet. Gynec.* 26: 1–8.

WORLD HEALTH ORGANIZATION. 1966. "Congenital malformations: A report of a study of series of consecutive births in 24 centres." *Bull. WHO,* Suppl., 34: 22–23.

YANNET, H. 1956. "Mental deficiency." *Adv. Pediat.* 8: 217–57.

ZELLWEGER, H. 1966. "Familial chromosomal aberrations. Part I—Introduction." *Ann. Paed.* 206: 317–32.

———. 1966. "Familial chromosomal aberrations. Part II—Familial aneuploides, mainly familial trisomies with karyotypically normal parents." *Ann. Paed.* 206: 381–95.

———. 1966. "Indications for chromosomal analysis in mongolism." *J. Iowa Med. Soc.* 56: 1221–26.

ZELLWEGER, H., ABBO, G., and CUANY, R. 1966. "Satellite association and translocation mongolism." *J. Med. Genet.* 3: 186–89.

Index

Abortions: chromosomal abnormalities in, 19, 22, 59; induced, 19; spontaneous, 19; and maternal age, 21; and maternal reproductive history, 60–61, 64; and maternal factors, 60, 62
Ages: of mongols, 104–5
Aging, 109; and meiotic accidents, 38
Androgyny scores, 70
Atmospheric temperature, 57
Australia antigen, 102
Autoimmunity, 71. *See* Thyroid antibodies

Birth certificates, 22, 38, 42
Birth control, 33, 43–44, 81
Bloom's Syndrome, 92

Chromatin: anomalies of sex, 58
Chromosome breaks, 2, 38, 93; and infectious hepatitis, 55; and viruses, 58
Chromosomes, 2; and abortions, 19, 22, 59; and radiation, 65; XXX females, 81; XXXXY males, 81; satellited, 108; types and etiology, 110
Chromosomes abnormal, 9, 78; types by race, 25–26; and infectious hepatitis, 55; and seasonal distribution, 57; and mycoplasma, 72; and familial aggregation, 75–79, 81; and twins, 83; and environmental agents, 92; and malignancies, 93; and thyroid antibodies, 95–96; and maternal age, 107
Coitus: frequency of, 37
Conceptions: frequency of trisomy 21 in, 21, 92
Congenital heart disease, 48, 98, 111; and mortality of mongols, 105
Congenital malformations, 111; incidence of, 23; clustering, 48; seasonal pattern, 56–57; prenatal factors, 59; radiation, 66; and thyroid antibodies, 72; in mice, 76
Consanguinity, 80–81, 108

Dental caries, 69
Dermatoglyphic surveys: percent of chromosomal mosaics, 9, 108
Diagnostic criteria: influence on incidence, 19, 23–24, 48
Dimethylbenzanthracene, 92

Endocrine factors, 59, 70, 94–96, 100–2; and nondisjunction, 108. *See* Thyroid antibodies; Thyroid disease
Environmental factors, 22, 38, 47, 109–10; and variability of mongols, 102, 111. *See* Etiological hypotheses; Radiation exposure

Enzyme studies, 100–2
Epidemiology, 22, 107–13; definition of, 9; demographic factors, 9. *See* Prospective studies; Retrospective studies
Ethnic factors, 22–26, 112
Etiological hypotheses: racial, 1; and epidemiology, 9; and environmental factors, 22; and radiation exposure, 66–68; and fluorides in water supply, 69–70

Familial aggregation, 75–84, 108
Fanconi's Syndrome, 92
Fertility, 59–64
Fertilization: delayed, 36–37
Fetal loss, 21–22, 59–65, 99
Furfuraceous idiocy, 1

Genetic factors, 22, 75–84, 93–94, 100, 104
Geographical areas, 47, 52, 57, 112
Gynecological disorders, 69

Harelip and cleft palate, 48, 66
Hirschsprung's disease, 98

Incidence, 47; definition of, 9–10
Infectious hepatitis, 50–51, 54–56, 102–3

Klinefelter's Syndrome, 38, 81, 97

Leucocytes, 91–92
Leukemia, 85–93; and radiation, 65, 92; and Australia antigen, 102

Marriage: age at, 63; number of, 73; duration of, 37, 60, 73
Maternal age, 10, 15, 21, 23–24, 27, 31; and birth order, 4, 28; and abortions, 21; and paternal age, 28, 39; and statistical analysis, 28–29; and bimodality, 29; independent–dependent, 29, 32, 108–9; birth control, 33; cytological types, 33–35; etiology, 35–38, 107, 110; reproductive performance, 62–63; recurrence risk, 76; familial aggregation, 77; and twinning, 84; thyroid antibodies, 96; oocyte deterioration, 108–9; risk factors, 109
Maternal factors: and incidence, 19, 59–74, 108
Meiosis, 2, 38, 59, 108
Mitosis, 9; and delayed fertilization, 36
Mosaics, 2, 71, 81, 108, 110; and frequency, 9; and grandmother's age, 42
Mycoplasma, 72–73

Newborns: methods to determine incidence among, 15; frequency of trisomy 21 among, 19
Nondisjunction, 2, 108–9; and maternal age, 35; and uterine selection, 35; chromosomal breaks, 37–38; atmospheric temperature, 57; fetal loss, 63; radiation, 65, 92; genetic factors, 80–81; secondary, 107–8

Ova: abnormal, 9, 36–38

Physical signs: variability of, 100, 111
Pregnancy free interval, 60, 64–65
Prevalence: definition of, 9–10
Prospective studies, 13

Radar exposure, 68
Radiation exposure, 65–68, 108
Recurrence risk, 42, 75–76, 78–79. *See* Maternal age
Respiratory infections, 104–5
Retrospective studies, 13, 23, 48
Rubella, 55

Sibs: frequency of mongols among, 75–76, 80; frequency of leukemia among, 89, 93–94
Socioeconomic status, 58
Statistical aspects, 40–41, 48, 52–56
Stillbirths. *See* Fetal loss
Streptococcal infections, 48
Survivorship, 104–6

Thyroid antibodies, 55, 71–72, 95–96; and maternal age, 96; and mosaic and translocation mongols, 96

Thyroid disease, 71, 94–96
Translocations: and familial aggregation, 2, 34, 76, 78, 80, 108, 110; reciprocal, 2; Negroes, 25; sporadic, 34; and maternal age, 39, 77, 107; paternal age, 39–40; frequency of, 40; thyroid disease, 71; maternal carrier, 78–79; inherited, 79; enzymes, 100. *See* Familial aggregation
Trisomy, 9, 108, 110–11; and familial factors, 76; enzymes, 100; and congenital heart disease, 111
Trisomy 13–15, 81
Trisomy 17–18, 81
Trisomy 21, 2; frequency among and spontaneous abortions, 19; incidence in conceptions, 21–22; and thyroid disease, 71; and mosaicism, 81
Turner's Syndrome, 81

Urban-rural areas, 10, 47–48, 50
Uterine bleeding: during pregnancy, 68–69
Uterine selection, 35–36

Viruses, 38, 50, 108; and chromosomal abnormalities, 58, 96; and familial aggregation, 81

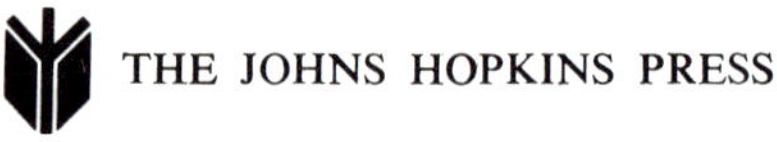

Designed by Arlene J. Sheer

Composed in Times Roman text and display
by Baltimore Type & Composition Corp.

Printed on 60-lb. Perkins and Squier R
by Universal Lithographers, Inc.

Bound in Columbia Milbank Vellum
by L. H. Jenkins Co., Inc.